# Total Care of the Lower Limb Amputee

# Total Care of the Lower Limb Amputee

**Ian M Troup,** MB, ChB, DMed Rehab
Consultant in Rehabilitation, Dundee Limb Fitting Centre
Senior Lecturer, Department of Orthopaedics, University of Dundee

**Marjorie A Wood,** MBE, SRN, SCM, HV, QNCert
Nursing Officer
Dundee Limb Fitting Centre

**Pitman**

PITMAN BOOKS LIMITED
128 Long Acre, London WC2E 9AN

PITMAN PUBLISHING INC.
1020 Plain Street, Marshfield, Massachusetts

*Associated Companies*
Pitman Publishing Pty Ltd, Melbourne
Pitman Publishing New Zealand Ltd, Wellington
Copp Clark Pitman, Toronto

First Published 1982

British Library Cataloguing in Publication Data

Troup, I. M.
Total care of the lower limb amputee.
1. Amputations of leg
2. Amputees—Rehabilitation
I. Title II. Wood, A. M.
362.4'3 RD560

ISBN 0-272-79641-7



Text set in 10/12 pt. Linotron 202 Times, printed and bound in Great Britain at The Pitman Press, Bath

This book is dedicated
to the International Year for
Disabled People and to the
continuing success in years
to come of work initiated
in 1981.

19 81

International Year of
Disabled People

*The logo for the International Year of Disabled People, 1981 represents two people holding hands in solidarity and support of each other in a position of equality. It reflects equality, hope and support. The leaves around the logo show part of the United Nations emblem.*

UNITED NATIONS

# Contents

*Dedication* v
*Foreword* ix
*Acknowledgements* x
**1** History 1
**2** Anatomy—Applied 6
**3** Bioengineering Principles and Human Locomotion 17
**4** Indications for Amputation 24
**5** Levels and Limiting Factors in Amputation Surgery 34
**6** Preoperative Care 40
**7** Significant Features of Amputation Surgery 47
**8** Postoperative Care 52
**9** Stump Dressings 61
**10** The Stump—Function and Associated Problems 76
**11** Prosthetic Replacement 80
**12** Technical Amputee Care 90
**13** Abnormalities of Amputee Gait 99
**14** Physiotherapy 104
**15** Rehabilitation in Activities of Daily Living (ADL) 118
**16** Feelings, Failings, and Frustrations 125
*Glossary of Terms* 128
*Bibliography* 131
*Index* 132

# Foreword

This book fills a gap in the literature. It may not be unique but there are few which attempt to approach the management of the amputee in this particular way.

The book is born of an experience which again if not unique is, at least, unusual. Both authors are founder members of a close knit clinic team dedicated to the care of the amputee. Both contributed in a substantial and significant way to a service which received international recognition. In writing this volume that experience comes over to the reader in the confidence of their opinions, in the detail of their practice and the assured display of knowledge of disciplines different from their own. As such it presents the most comprehensive description of the sequence of events and the essential elements in the care of the amputee available today.

The volume brings out in a most vivid way the role of the different professionals involved. It will demonstrate that the most informed and the most dexterous exercise of the key roles of surgeon and prosthetist will not, in itself, ensure a satisfactory outcome.

The authors are to be congratulated on producing a volume which will not only provide the medical student, the nurse, and therapist in training an insight into the treatment of the amputee but also illuminate many aspects of the concept of rehabilitation. So far as the professionals are concerned, be they prosthetic technicians, prosthetists, nurses, doctors, therapists, surgeons, or administrators this volume should be compulsory reading.

My hope is that it will find a wide distribution amongst the professions because I am convinced that it will thereby bring about an improved level of care and increased harmony within the professionals.

George Murdoch

Professor of Orthopaedic Surgery
and Traumatology,
University of Dundee.

# Acknowledgements

It would have been impossible to compile this book without the experience of working in a unit devoted to amputee care. The authors wish to recognise the professionalism and dedication of the staff and in particular wish to thank Mrs Marilyn Copland for her secretarial help and Miss Margaret Sturrock for her work on the illustrations.

# 1 History

The loss of a limb appears to date back to prehistoric times. It seems certain that congenitally limb deficient children have been one of humanity's problems throughout history. Ancient mosaics and pottery indicate the use of prosthetic devices in the form of wooden peg legs and supporting crutches from as early as the Gallo-Roman era. The earliest known prosthetic device was recovered from a tomb and dates back to 300 BC. In a sense, the materials used in those days differed very slightly from those in use in more recent years—wood and copper were used in ancient times and wood is still used in certain countries, although copper is no longer the metal of choice. The prosthetic devices were mainly primitive and reminiscent of that used by R L Stevenson's character, Long John Silver. The more elaborate prostheses were only used by knights and warriors of ancient times. Those were fabricated by the armourers and were largely intended to conceal limb loss suffered in battle.

Surgical practice in amputation has varied. Hippocrates understood the use of ligatures but for many centuries bleeding was controlled by crushing the stump and dipping it in boiling oil. Hans von Gersdoff (floruit 1490–1520) advocated the use of warm, not boiling oil as a dressing and covering the stump with a flap of skin and muscle. Ligatures were again used by Ambroise Paré, a French army surgeon, in the first half of the sixteenth century. Amputation was, as a result, more frequently used as a life saving measure especially by surgeons in the field. The rate of survival increased with the improved control of haemorrhage and later, towards the end of the seventeenth century, Morel introduced the use of the tourniquet, resulting in further improvement in technique. Dominique Jean Larrey (1766–1842), Napoleon's personal surgeon, tried refrigeration to dull the pain of amputation. At this time amputation was the commonest of all surgical procedures. It was therefore natural that Paré and others should interest themselves in the production of a prosthesis for what was usually an above-knee limb loss, and development reached even the introduction of artificial joints. It is interesting to note that the artificial limbs bore a strong resemblance to the armour worn by the knights of those times. The prostheses produced late in the seventeenth century by another surgeon, Verduin, for below-knee limb loss, bear a remarkable resemblance in design to those used by some amputees in modern times. They were the first devices to allow free use of the knee.

The next advance was in the use of wood instead of the heavier metals by James Potts of London in 1800. The socket for the above-knee stump was fashioned in wood, the knee joints were made of steel and the foot was articulated. Even at this early date an attempt was made to introduce artificial tendons to operate the ankle and foot, the motor force being the movement of the knee joint. This resulted in the foot being held up when the knee was flexed, thereby easing the swing-through of the leg. This limb became known as the Anglesey limb since it was worn by the Marquis of Anglesey after he lost his leg at Waterloo. This type of limb was finally used and developed in America and fitted to many soldiers after the American Civil War. It was commercially available for 99 years, in fact until 1915. One such limb, made for the Marquis of Anglesey, along with his tattered Hussar trouser leg can be seen in the museum at Plas Newydd, Anglesey.

Some progress had thus been made in artificial limb design, and several events to come were to improve the surgical practice concerned with amputation. A functional stump evolved by design rather than by fortuitous circumstance.

An event of immense surgical importance was the discovery and use of chloroform by Dr Simpson of Edinburgh in 1847. No longer was it necessary to remove a limb in seconds with the patient, if he was lucky, in a totally inebriated condition. The use of anaesthetics allowed care to be taken and amputation stumps literally took shape. However, the increased surgical intervention led to increased infection, and it was only later in the 1860s, following Louis Pasteur's recognition of the cause of infection, and Lord Lister's discovery of the method for controlling infection with carbolic acid, that further progress was made.

Lister's statistics are of considerable interest (see Table 1.1). These advances—chloroform and the control of infection—resulted in a reduced mortality following major amputation surgery from 50% to 10%.

**Table 1.1**

| | *Total cases* | *Recovered* | *Died* |
|---|---|---|---|
| Prior to control of infection | 35 | 19 (54.3%) | 16 (45.7%) |
| Following control of infection | 40 | 34 (85%) | 6 (15%) |

It must already be clear that major wars, although causing grief and sorrow, produced the necessary stimulus in new techniques and prosthetic design. Following the 1914–18 and 1939–45 wars great advances were made and, more recently, Korea and Vietnam, with the devastating effect of modern weaponry involved, focused opinion and aid on those unfortunate enough to lose a limb.

It is strange that modern medicine has produced its own problem in this field. By virtue of the fact that much of the amputation surgery prior to this century was necessitated by injury, most of the patients were relatively young. As people live longer, and particularly since the inception of intensive geriatric care, the limb-deficient patient of advancing years is becoming more and more a clinical entity. This may result, at least in part, from changing ways of life in the Western world. Views are now held, not without good foundation, associating atherosclerosis, the disease commonly preceding amputation, with the way of life and habits of the people of Europe and the North American continent.

It is worthwhile mentioning that in 1948 (Figure 1.1) when the United

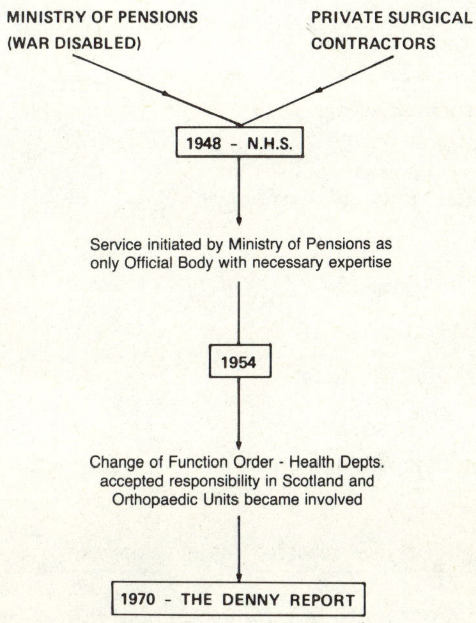


**Figure 1.1** The development of a limb service from 1948 to 1970

Kingdom National Health Service was born, there was no artificial limb service other than that supplied by the Ministry of Pensions for ex-servicemen and since it became necessary to provide treatment for patients of all ages, clearly the existing services could not now deal with the age groups involved. This led, in Scotland, to the artificial limb service coming within the administrative structure of the Regional Hospital Boards in the early 1950s. It was inevitable that this should result in comment and criticism by hospital staffs regarding the adequacy of the provisions for the amputee. Fortunately this formed constructive appraisal and has produced beneficial results.

More recently, in 1970, the Scottish Home and Health Department produced a report on the Future of the Artificial Limb Service in Scotland. Popularly known as the Denny Report* this visualised a further improvement in the care of the amputee (Table 1.2). It suggested that intensive

**Table 1.2 Clinic team**

| | |
|---|---|
| Training programmes—Prosthetist : leading to professional status | |
| —Doctor : courses and in-service training | |
| Limb fitting surgeon involvement prior to operation | |
| In patient units for amputee care | |
| Doctor/patient contact to be more adequate | |
| Modular limb assembly systems | |
| Rapid limb delivery and rehabilitation | |
| Adequate patient training in limb use | |
| Linkage with orthotic services research and development | |

care amputee inpatient units be established, and that associated with these units there should be all the necessary prosthetic expertise in the shape of highly skilled prosthetists, backed up by trained technicians and all the

* The Future of the Artificial Limb Service in Scotland. (SHHD 1970) 'Denny Working Party Report'.

'Those concerned with the treatment of the amputees, from amputation to re-training for employment when necessary should work together as a clinic team, each being of professional status and playing his part in the patient's rehabilitation.'

'Patients should ideally be transferred to the charge of the prosthetic surgeon before amputation and have the operation carried out by him.'

'The proper fitting and quick delivery of artificial limbs is of paramount importance.'

'Patients need thorough training appropriate to their needs in using their artificial limbs.'

'All limb-fitting centres should have beds associated with them.'

equipment and materials necessary. There should be paramedical expertise and, most important of all, there should be available nursing and therapy skills of a high order. The aim of these specialised units must be total care, and at long last it appears that the care of the amputee will reach a more acceptable level. It was by design that the Scottish system developed and, although in England the Artificial Limb Service remained a Ministry responsibility, much progress has been made. However if the concepts of Denny are believed, Health Department responsibility must be achieved. The limb fitting surgeon is a clinician and much is gained by a clinical association with colleagues involved in many ways in amputee care.

Throughout the world there is great variation in modern prosthetic practice—many factors are involved—presenting pathology, financial implications, the presence or absence of state-planned health care, to mention but a few. The variation also involves materials, fabrication, and what may be recognised as expertise specifically associated with certain countries. Centres of excellence have developed such as are seen in Scandinavia and elsewhere in Europe. The United States of America has injected large sums of money and research and development work has advanced rapidly. This worldwide interest has come together in the shape of the International Society for Prosthetics and Orthotics. Exchange of information, education, and training are developing throughout the world with considerable benefit to the amputee. Much work remains to be done, and the importance of each professional team member within this field must never be underestimated. In keeping with certain other areas of the caring professions, this is a specialised field offering considerable satisfaction in what must be a very real human problem.

# 2 Anatomy—Applied

This is a subject which, when considered against the pattern of bipedal human gait, is soon found to be immensely complicated. It is not the intention in this chapter to study anatomy in depth, but it is hoped that it will lead to a basic appreciation of what is involved.

Various studies of muscle activity in the lower limb whilst walking have been made, and it is clear that approximately 30 individual muscles in each leg can be involved in simply taking one step forward. These muscles can be classified as having particular functions: amongst other things, a shock absorbing and a torso balancing action (Table 2.1). It must be remembered that during normal gait the trunk and the upper limbs are involved, and muscle groups throughout the whole body are active whilst walking. There must, of course, be added to this, coordination and timing to produce a normal pattern of gait. It is in this context that pure applied anatomy can conveniently be described.

It is useful to look upon the lower limbs as pillars supporting the torso above, and exerting forces on the ground below. However, these pillars are jointed and the joints, although necessary for normal gait, need to be controlled. This control is effected by various muscle groups and tendons, the extent of the control depending on their power and the characteristics of each joint. It should be remembered that muscles have three particular types of action or activity:

1. they perform motor work, in other words they flex and extend joints;
2. they act almost like the guy ropes of a tent and stabilise joints in certain positions;
3. they act as shock absorbers and in this context it will be appreciated that if a muscle is to act as a shock absorber it tends to lengthen or stretch, but even in this situation it is still doing work.

It is necessary to consider each joint individually.

## The hip

The hip (Figure 2.1) is a ball and socket joint and naturally allows movement in all directions—flexion, extension, abduction, adduction, and rotation. All these movements are necessary to a varying degree when walking, if the pattern is to be normal. This will be appreciated more fully in later chapters. However, it can be seen that several muscles and muscle groups are involved in order to introduce the necessary controlled function. They are, in the main (Figures 2.2 and 2.3):

| | |
|---|---|
| Flexors: | psoas<br>rectus femoris<br>sartorius |
| Extensors: | gluteus maximus<br>hamstrings<br>adductor magnus (partly)<br>gluteus medius (partly) |
| Abductors: | gluteus medius<br>gluteus minimus<br>tensor fasciae latae |
| Adductors: | the three adductors (longus, brevis, magnus)<br>gluteus maximus (partly) |
| Medial rotators: | gluteus medius } anterior fibres<br>gluteus minimus } anterior fibres |
| Lateral rotators: | pectineus<br>psoas<br>gluteus maximus—lower fibres<br>quadratus femoris |

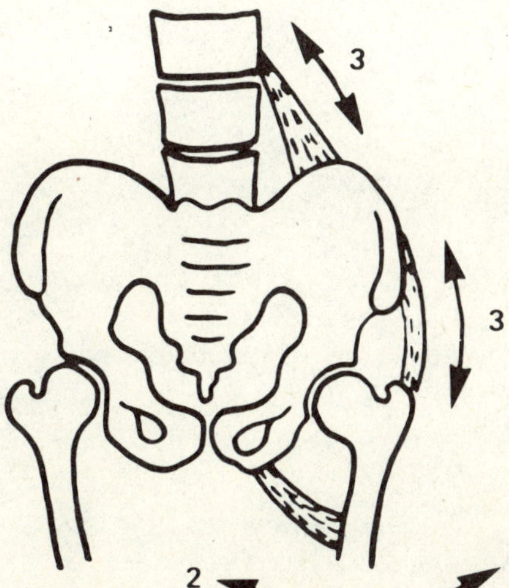


**Figure 2.1** Around the hip as well as flexion, extension, and rotation, there is abduction (1), adduction (2), and control of trunk stabilisation (3)

This muscle action and resulting hip function is complicated even further by seeing some muscles acting in a dual capacity—the adductors as hip flexors and the abductors mainly serving as torso balancers. Finally it must be recognised that body posture can vary muscle action—the psoas is a flexor of the hip joint and a medial rotator of the thigh until flexion is almost complete when it becomes a lateral rotator.

## The knee joint

The knee joint (Figure 2.4) is quite different, being basically a swivel joint

**Table 2.1 Classification of muscles by function**

| |
|---|
| *Shock absorbers* |
| Vastus intermedius |
| Vastus lateralis |
| Vastus medialis |
| Rectus femoris |
| *Torso balancers* |
| Gluteus maximus |
| Gluteus medius |
| Gluteus minimus |
| Tensor fasciae latae |
| Erector spinae |
| *Push off group* |
| Flexor digitorum longus |
| Flexor hallucis longus |
| Gastrocnemius |
| Peroneus brevis |
| Peroneus longus |
| Soleus |
| Tibialis posterior |
| *Accelerators hip flexion* |
| Adductor longus |
| Adductor magnus |
| Iliacus (iliopsoas) |
| Sartorius |
| *Foot flexion shock absorbers at time of heel strike* |
| Extensor digitorum longus |
| Extensor hallucis longus |
| Tibialis anterior |
| *Decelerators. Hamstrings* |
| Gracilis |
| Semimembranosus |
| Semitendinosus |
| Biceps femoris (long head) |
| Biceps femoris (short head) |

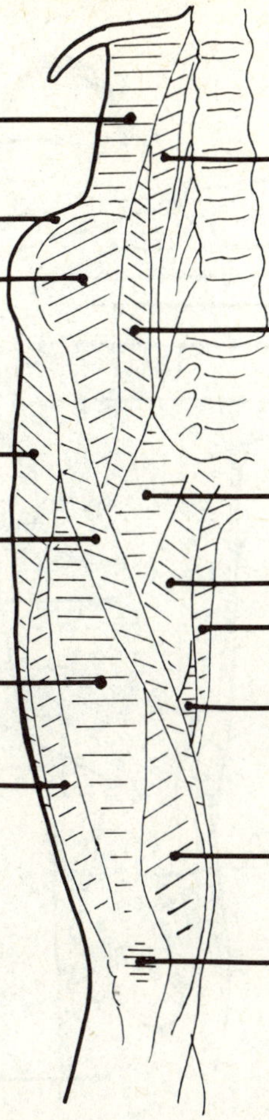


**Figure 2.2** The hip, anterior view

with one plane of action—flexion and extension. It is a large joint highly dependent on powerful ligaments and muscles. Any movement in an anteroposterior or lateral plane indicates laxity of supporting ligaments, but a certain amount of rotation is possible and does take place during normal gait. Flexion and extension of the knee are controlled by (Figures 2.5 and 2.6):

Flexors: biceps femoris
popliteus
sartorius
semitendinosus
semimembranosus

Extensors: the four parts of the quadriceps femoris

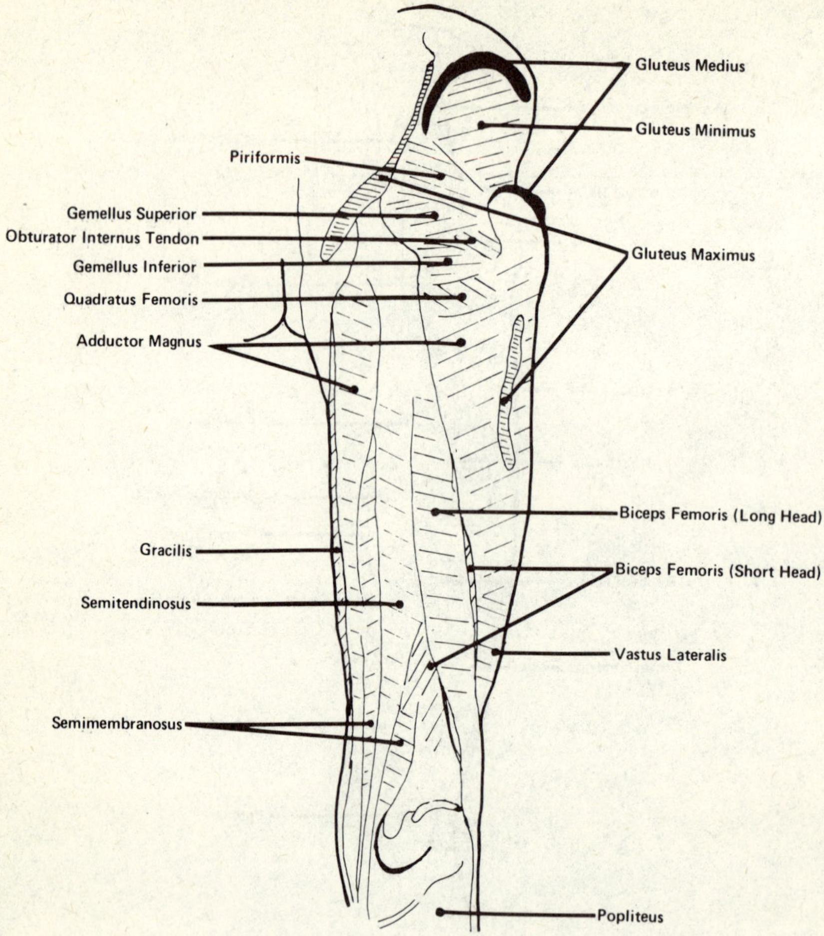


**Figure 2.3** The hip, posterior view

Flexion is normally limited by soft tissue resistance between the calf and thigh. Extension is limited by the anterior cruciate ligament, the medial and lateral ligaments, and the posterior joint capsule. In the latter situation the knee is firmly locked, in the former it is lax and rotation can occur. The rotators are:

Medial rotators: popliteus
gracilis
sartorius
semitendinosus
semimembranosus
Lateral rotator: biceps femoris

It is interesting that some of these muscles have a dual function, being two

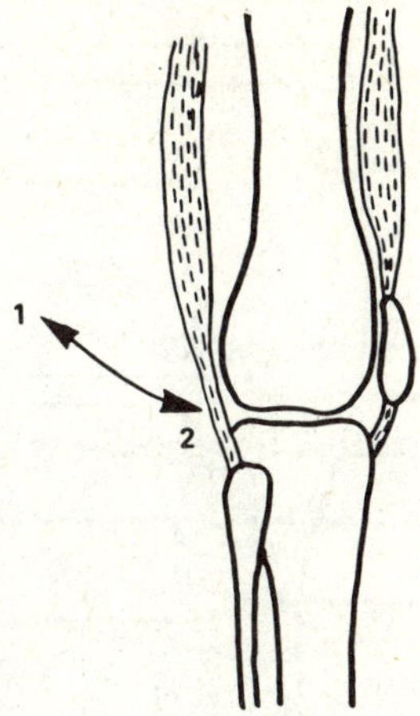


**Figure 2.4** At the knee there is flexion (1) and extension (2)

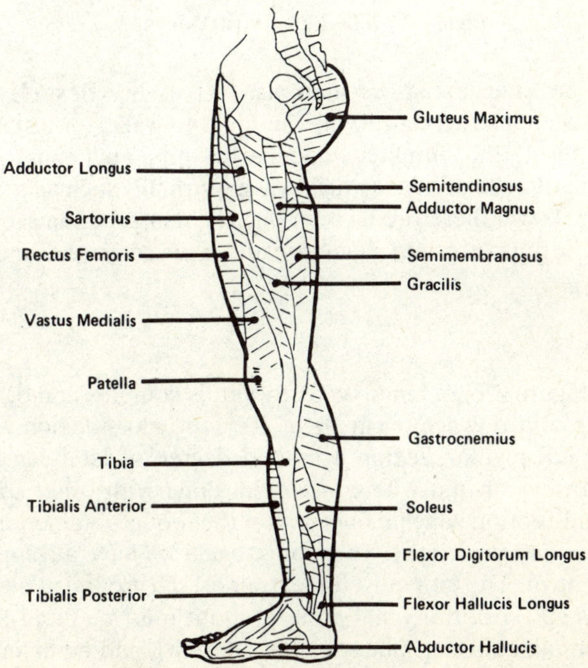


**Figure 2.5** The knee, medial view

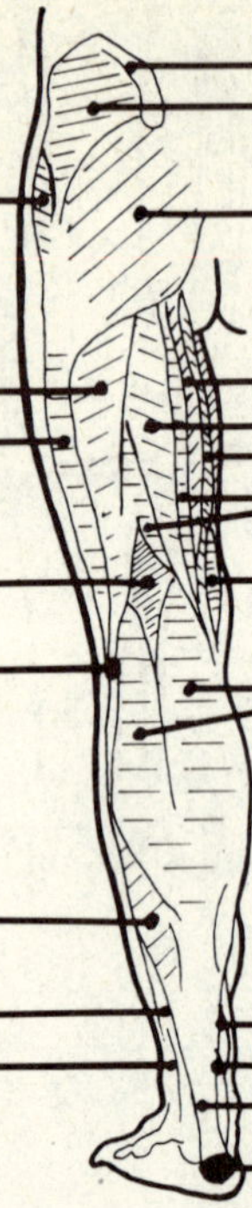


**Figure 2.6** The knee, posterior view

joints, i.e. the knee extensors may also act as hip flexors. This is of importance when instructing certain amputees to walk; for instance, in the above-knee level, the amputee extends his hip, and consequently his stump, in order to extend the artificial knee; normally such an action would flex the knee. It will therefore be seen that the control of an artificial knee may involve a muscle group diametrically opposed to the one normally used.

## The ankle

The ankle (Figure 2.7), a hinge type of joint, is complex and basically only allows an up and down movement of the foot (dorsiflexion and plantar flexion). In full plantar flexion a limited degree of lateral movement is possible. However it must be considered along with other joints in the hind- and mid-foot, in which movement of the foot is obtained from side to side (eversion and inversion). Thus, once again we have a complex system of muscle control. The foot must force itself off the ground at push off prior to taking a step (posterior tibial group), and it must be lifted to clear the ground when taking a step (anterior tibial group), and be maintained in a level position by controlling eversion and inversion (peroneals).

Dorsiflexion and plantar flexion of the ankle take place around a

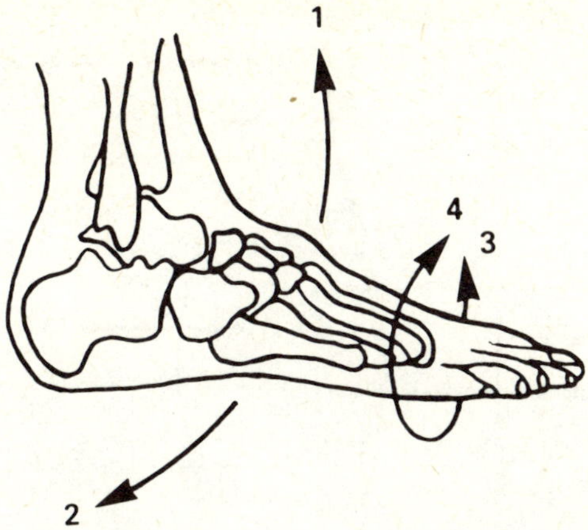


**Figure 2.7** At the ankle there is dorsiflexion (1) and plantar flexion (2) with inversion (3) and eversion (4) of the foot

horizontal axis which is not transverse, inclining backwards from the medial to the lateral side. The articular surfaces are broader anteriorly and the further dorsiflexion takes place, the firmer is the grip on the talus by the malleoli. In the erect position the talus is firmly held in the bony socket and since the load line of the centre of gravity is anteriorly placed, the joint is held firmly locked. However, in full plantar flexion as on tip-toe, there is limited lateral movement, the talus no longer being firmly locked in position. Stability is maintained by the:

Calcaneofibular band
Posterior talofibular band
Deltoid ligament
Posterior capsule
} in dorsiflexion

Anterior talofibular band
Anterior fibres deltoid ligament
Anterior capsule
} in plantar flexion

Dorsiflexion and plantar flexion are controlled by (Figures 2.8–2.10):

| | |
|---|---|
| Dorsiflexors: | tibialis anterior |
| | extensor digitorum longus |
| | extensor hallucis longus |
| | peroneus tertius |
| Plantar flexors: | gastrocnemius |
| | soleus |
| | plantaris |
| | tibialis posterior |
| | long flexors of the toes |
| | peroneus longus |
| | peroneus brevis |

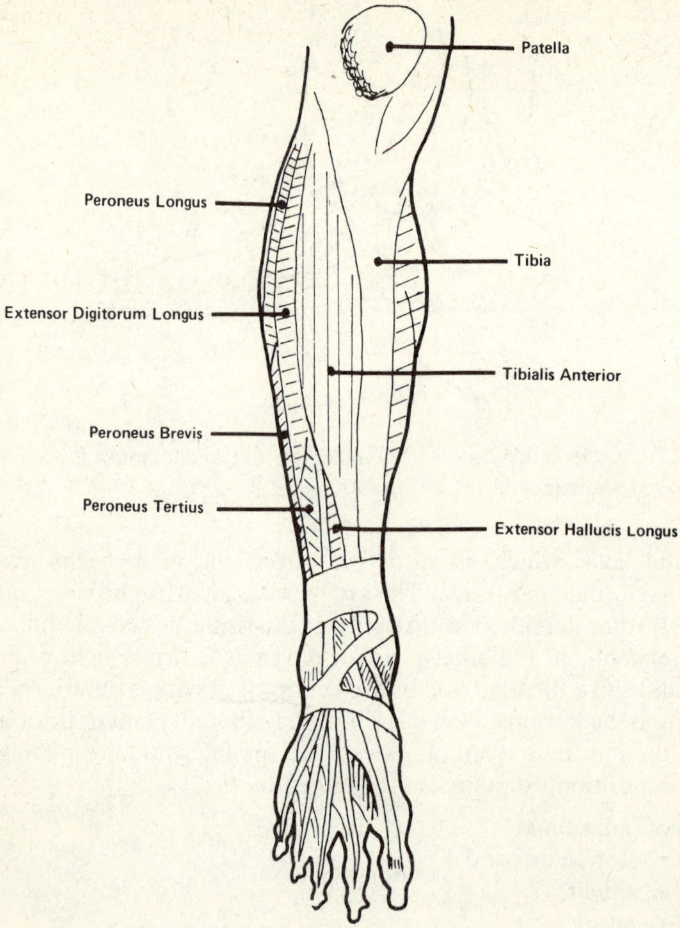


**Figure 2.8** The ankle, anterior view

## The forefoot

The forefoot must move in an up and down plane and rotate, its function being intimately connected with that of the ankle and hindfoot. Thus it will be seen that the whole foot/ankle complex tends to act, or should act, as one unit. The structure of the foot is complex, the many joints and ligaments having their own special significance. Of particular importance are the plantar calcaneonavicular ligament or 'spring' ligament and the long plantar ligament, both of which play an important part in maintaining the arch of the foot.

Finally, one should not forget that nearly all the muscles in the body are involved when walking, the trunk, the upper limbs, the head and neck. An

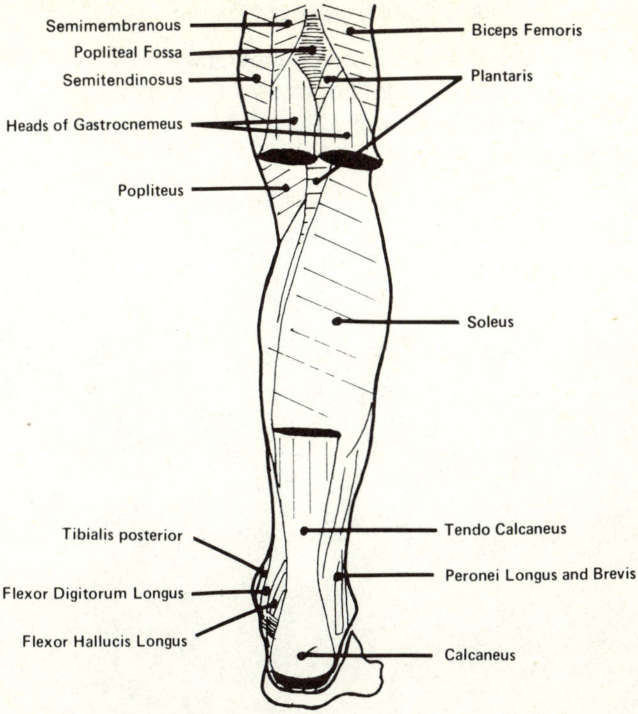


**Figure 2.9** The ankle, posterior view

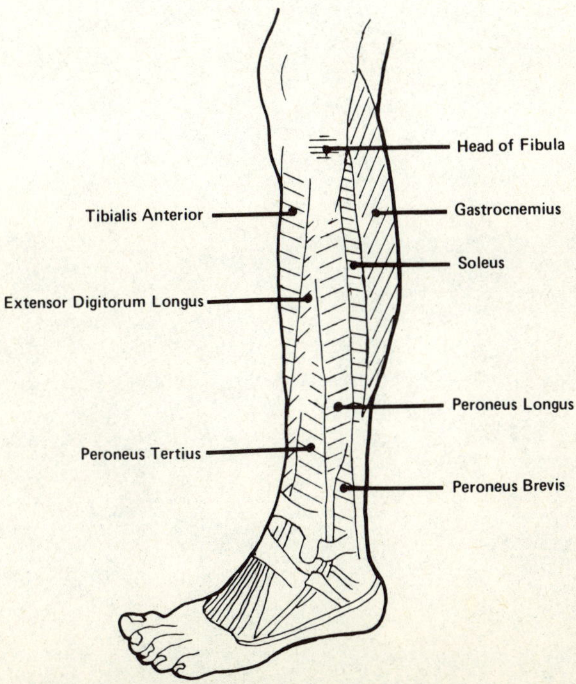


**Figure 2.10** The ankle, lateral view

individual walking purely with lower limb movement would look most unnatural and although we need not display the guardsman's precision we do require some upper body movement to produce a natural gait either purposeful or casual.

# 3 **Bioengineering Principles and Human Locomotion**

The disciplines and skills required in the care of the amputee necessitated an extension of the specialisation seen in medicine today. The bioengineer, an engineer with particular knowledge and ability to apply his skill in the medical field, is a new concept, as yet rarely seen in the hospital service in the United Kingdom. He frequently works behind the scenes producing ideas or hardware of use to the doctor. In the field of prosthetics his association with the patient must be direct—in effect he is half engineer and half doctor, and ideally should work closely with the doctor responsible for the patient's care. The value of the bioengineer should never be underestimated in prosthetic work. His skills are based on sound theory and basic engineering principles, and by the application of these he can define the problem, leaving the problems which cannot be dealt with in this way to his medical colleagues; it is for this reason that the doctor/bioengineer team in prosthetics is so valuable.

Certain bioengineering principles may seem too simple to mention, but they are basic to the understanding of human gait.

Biomechanics, one branch of bioengineering, is the study of mechanics as applied to the human body, mechanics being a subject dealing with forces and their effect (Figure 3.1).

*Force* is that which changes, or tends to change, a body's state of rest or motion. Kicking a football at the beginning of a game clearly changes its state of rest, and a tennis racket or a cricket bat changes, or should change, the state of motion of the ball.

You may wonder what this has to do with gait but when you realise that *gravity*, which governs all our movements, is simply a force, the connection becomes obvious.

Another term used by engineers is a *moment*. If, for instance, a wrestler forces his opponent's hand back and perhaps makes him bend his elbow, he is creating a bending moment around the elbow by the application of this force on the hand. This situation is always present when walking—for instance, the forces between the ground and the foot create a moment at the knee. This, of course, is overcome by a muscular response which counteracts the moment, and thus controls the movement of the joint.

One further term frequently considered is *energy*. It is basically the capacity for doing work, and in walking the work may be heavy or light. This in turn varies the energy expenditure of the individual.

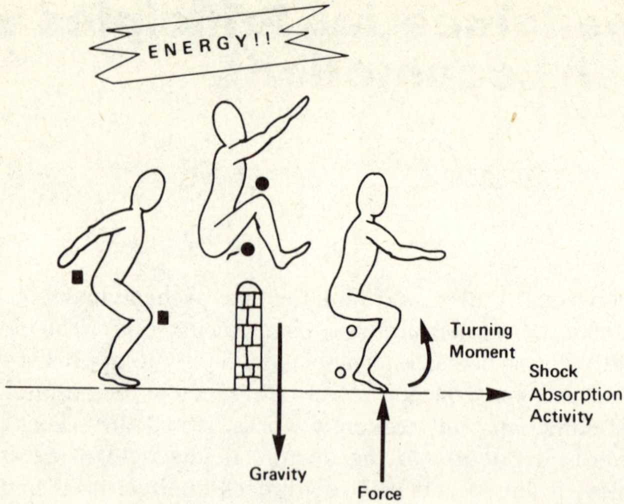


**Figure 3.1** Muscle activity: ■, performing motor work; ●, 'guy' wire activity—stabilisation; ○, shock absorbing

Thus we have several basic biomechanical terms to consider—*force*, *gravity*, *moment* and *energy*—all inter-related and clearly connected with human gait; simple ways of describing their application may be useful.

Consider a wheel or ball rolling on the ground (Figure 3.2)—a force is required to move it, but the centre of gravity of the wheel or ball only

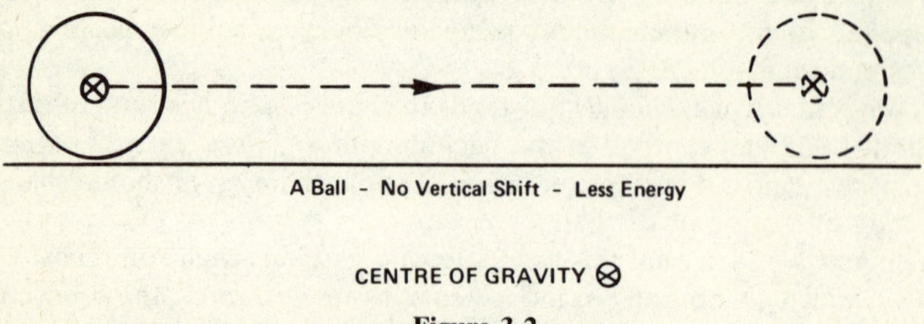


**Figure 3.2**

moves horizontally, there being no question of raising it against gravity or resisting the effect of gravity in a downwards direction, thus the energy requirement is low.

Next consider a man carrying a log and later trailing it (Figure 3.3). First he must lift it, thereby expending energy. After a few steps he finds it too heavy and must lower it to the ground. In doing so a moment is created around the knees, flexion having to be resisted. This is repeated several times and then, if the ground is smooth, he tries trailing the log, finding it much more effective and less tiring. This is entirely due to the fact that

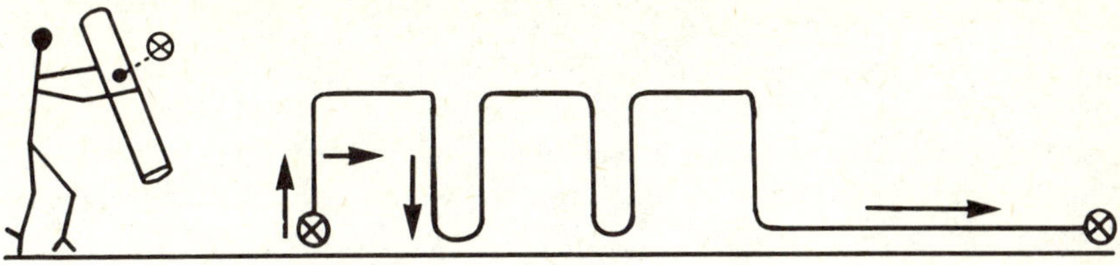


**Figure 3.3**

initially he must overcome or resist the force of gravity when lifting or lowering the log, and later, when trailing the log, this is no longer necessary.

Human gait can be seen to include all the aforementioned factors. We all have a centre of gravity—in effect just in front of the second sacral vertebral segment. We all must exert force to overcome gravity. Forces are exerted from the body above and the ground below, and moments are created around all the joints in the legs.

Finally, we all expend energy whilst walking, and it can now be seen that the energy requirement depends upon the forces applied and is directly related to the movement of the centre of gravity during gait. It is now necessary to describe how these basic bioengineering principles can be applied to human locomotion.

Since man appeared on our planet, whatever his origin, he has depended on his ability to move from one place to another. Some authorities believe that originally, like apes, we used a quadrupedal method of progression. Certainly for many thousands of years man has been a bipedal creature. Over the years his manner of gait has changed, largely due to external circumstances, but in the evolution of human gait a certain pattern has developed compatible with our present day existence.

Although this pattern has been achieved, it is difficult, indeed almost impossible, to define the state of normality. However, an attempt must be made to define normality if we are to be successful in recognising that which is seen, namely the abnormal pattern associated with general gait problems and in particular those concerning the amputee.

This subject of normality must be approached on a wide base line. There are so many factors involved in determining the pattern and only the most important will be mentioned in this publication. Some may be obvious, others less so. Clearly the body weight influences gait, as does the height and general stature of the individual. The mental attitude, if elevated, may impose a briskness on walking and, of course, the opposite similarly applies. Clothing can play an important part—fashion may demand a design which impedes walking, and naturally footwear, particularly heel height, changes the posture and the manner of gait. It is generally appreciated that frequently these factors cause pelvic contortions, invariably resulting in either pleasure or amusement, or indeed both. All these points are basically reflected in the length, width, and angle of each step. Finally, an over-riding element is the coordination of each step (Figure 3.4).

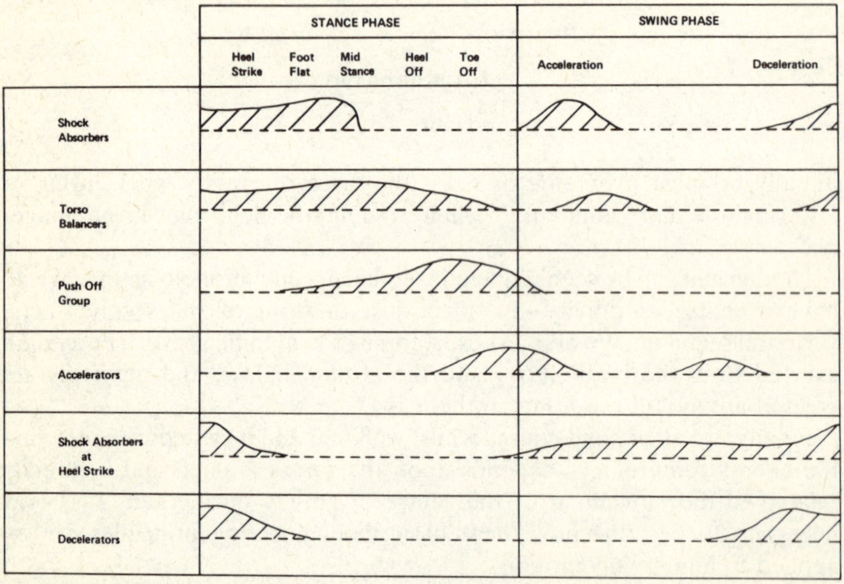


**Figure 3.4** Electromyographic activity

Normal gait can be broken down conveniently into certain specific cycles; each leg, in turn, goes through a stance phase and a swing phase. The stance phase is the period in which the leg is supporting the body weight, and the swing phase allows the leg to pass the other limb, which meantime is performing the weight bearing cycle of its own stance phase. Each phase has its own components.

1 Stance phase (Figure 3.5). Heel strike, the initiation of the stance phase, is the moment of impact, and fortunately the body is designed to absorb the force at this time. If it did not do so, every step would result in a jarring impact which would be felt all over the body. It performs this function by controlling the foot and ankle into the next part of the phase—mid stance. Clearly at this time the body weight is on this foot and the foot itself is flat on the ground. A little later, the heel rises and the toe exerts a push off which carries the foot through to the next phase.

2 Swing phase (Figure 3.6). This simply amounts to the toe leaving

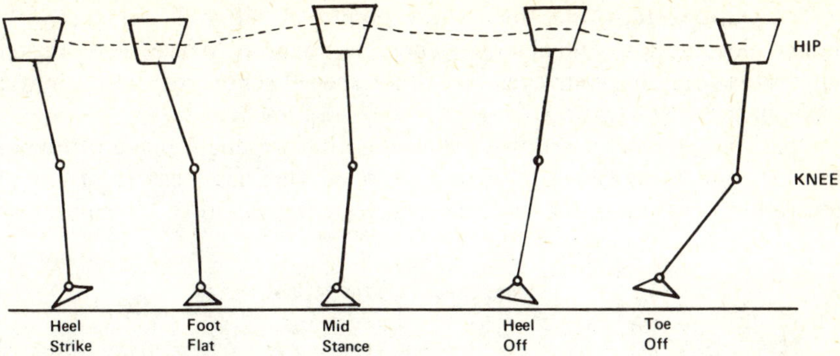


**Figure 3.5** Stance, high energy phase. Leg decelerated at heel strike; shock is absorbed at time of heel strike; torso is balanced at mid stance; motion is initiated at push off

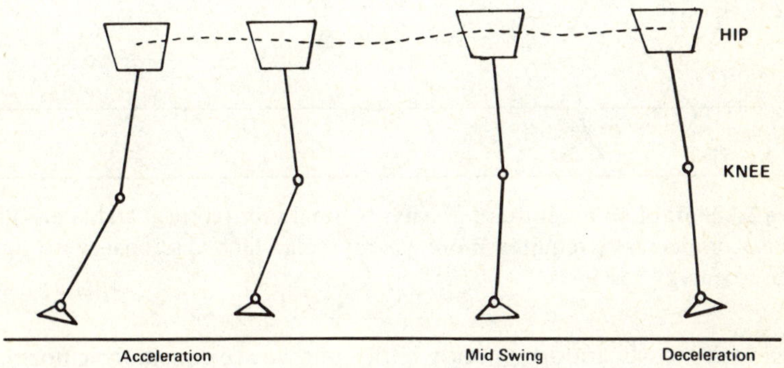


**Figure 3.6** Swing, low energy phase. Hip flexion initiated; knee extensors damp excess heel rise; toe dorsiflexed in mid swing; decelerating swing leg with hamstrings

the ground, the leg accelerating, clearing the walking surface and moving on once again to heel strike.

It should be remembered that all the joints in the lower limb are taking some part in this action. In brisk gait each foot goes through these phases about 55–60 times each minute and each leg must show coordinated movement within itself and with the other leg—a complex function for such a simple thing as taking a step.

It is interesting that the stance, or weight bearing phase uses more energy than the swing phase. During the stance phase, the effort of weight bearing is costly on energy. The swing phase, however, has a low energy cost, the main work being performed in slowing down the leg before heel strike, i.e. deceleration of the leg.

Take a few steps and study these points. A different perspective of human locomotion will emerge. There is no need to use sophisticated apparatus—rely on your eyes and other special senses, as did the physicians of the past.

There is a further worthwhile consideration we might make of human locomotion. As has already been mentioned man has a centre of gravity located just in front of the second sacral vertebra (Figure 3.7)—naturally it

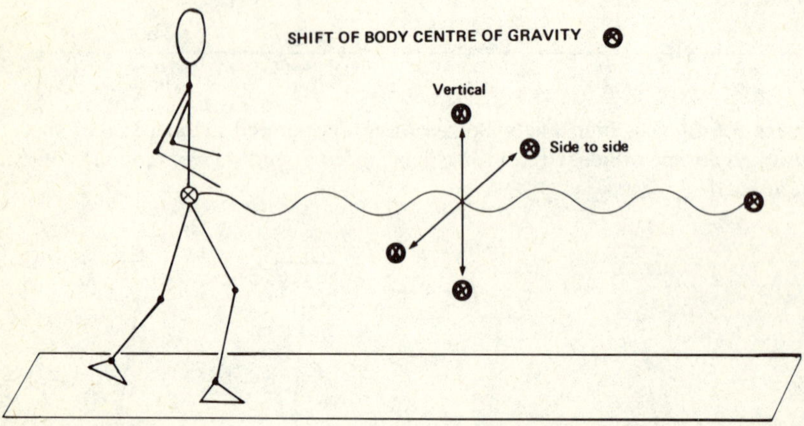


**Figure 3.7** Shift of body centre of gravity. Normal shift (vertical and lateral) 5 cm. Increase or decrease requires more energy (e.g. limb discrepancy = limp = increased energy cost)

varies with grossly abnormal body build, but we are considering normality. This centre of gravity, quite naturally, moves when we walk. Like any other solid object with a centre of gravity, energy is expended in starting the body moving and in stopping it from moving. Further, we can see that it must move from side to side as each foot in turn is in the stance phase. It also moves up and down to some degree as we walk, which may perhaps be less obvious. We can say therefore that when we are walking our centres of gravity move in the line of progression from side to side, up and down, each movement having to be initiated and, in turn, stopped and reversed. All of this amounts to work done—why? You can refer back to the last chapter and recall the basic physics. In order to start any body motion or, indeed, to change its course, or stop it, work must be done.

Why should all this emphasis be placed on what seems so very obvious? It is an attempt to show that normal gait, as opposed to abnormal gait described in a later chapter, does not expend too much energy. Any departure can be tiring and costly in energy consumption. The little boy or girl hurrying beside his parent and walking outwith his normal pattern soon gets tired. The small soldier keeping up with his taller companions also tires readily.

Why should this happen when we depart from a normal pattern? Remember the centre of gravity and its movement; associate this with the person's body weight, perhaps even as much as 90 kg or more, and finally carry out a simple estimation of how tiring it would be to move this weight each time a step is taken, indeed 110–120 times every minute whilst walking.

# 4 **Indications for Amputation**

The indications can conveniently be grouped and listed as follows:

1 vascular disease,
2 tumour,
3 trauma or injury,
4 chronic infection,
5 paralysis, deformity, and limb discrepancy,
6 congenital limb deficiency.

## Vascular disease

Vascular disease, or atherosclerosis, is a condition showing a worldwide variation in incidence. It is a disease of the more developed countries and is therefore commonly seen in northern America and Europe. The authors' experience suggests that over 60% of all primary amputees, that is those suffering limb loss for the first time, fall into this group. It appears to be associated directly with standards and mode of living and longer life expectancy. A further 28% have diabetes mellitus with associated vascular disease (Figure 4.1).

The incidence of vascular disease in amputation surgery warrants a brief comment on the pathology. Arterial blockage is caused by:

1 a degenerative condition of the vessel called atheroma;
2 thrombus formation in the vessel, thought to be secondary to the atheroma;
3 embolic impaction from another source, e.g. cardiac.

There are three coats in the wall of an artery—the intima, or internal coat, the media which is mainly muscle, and the externa forming a firmer outer coat. Atheroma of the vessel causes a thickening and rigidity of the intima with the deposition of fat and general friability of the tissues. When the atheroma is heaped up it forms plaques with narrowing of the lumen of the vessel. This in turn causes turbulence in the blood flow and the formation of a thrombus. In addition, the muscle coat of the vessel loses its pliability, rupturing easily and perhaps calcifying.

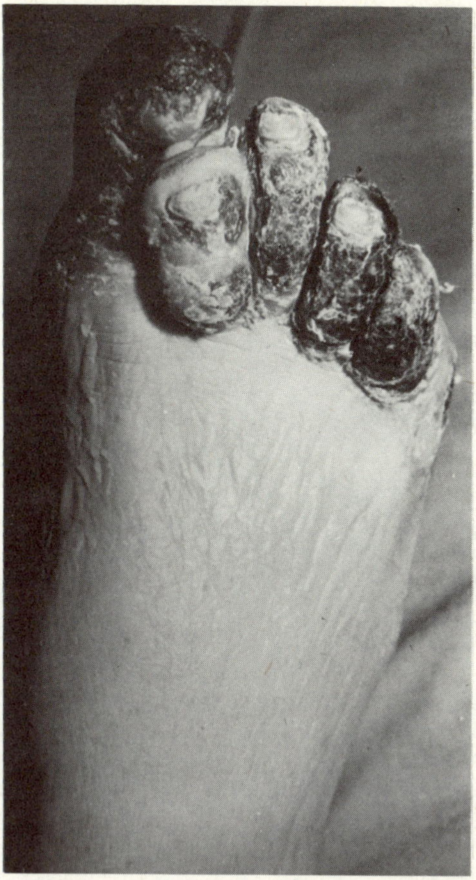

**Figure 4.1** Forefoot changes in advanced vascular disease

Atheroma is associated with areas of the vascular bed of high mean pressure—the distal vessels, because of this, are relatively free. It is also associated with high plasma cholesterol levels which are seen in conditions like diabetes, nephrotic syndrome, and hypertension. There is also a clear association with obesity and some non-vegetable foods.

It should not be forgotten that atheroma is a generalised disease and may result in conditions other than, or as well as, limb loss, e.g. myocardial infarction, cerebrovascular accident (CVA), renal failure, etc. There is also the question of the disease affecting the remaining leg in single amputees and resulting in rest or claudicating pain (Figure 4.2).

It is fitting at this point to mention the surgical problem of deciding the level of amputation discussed in a following chapter. Generally speaking, the more distal the level (in atherosclerosis), the greater is the severity of the disease. At the same time it must be remembered that the higher the

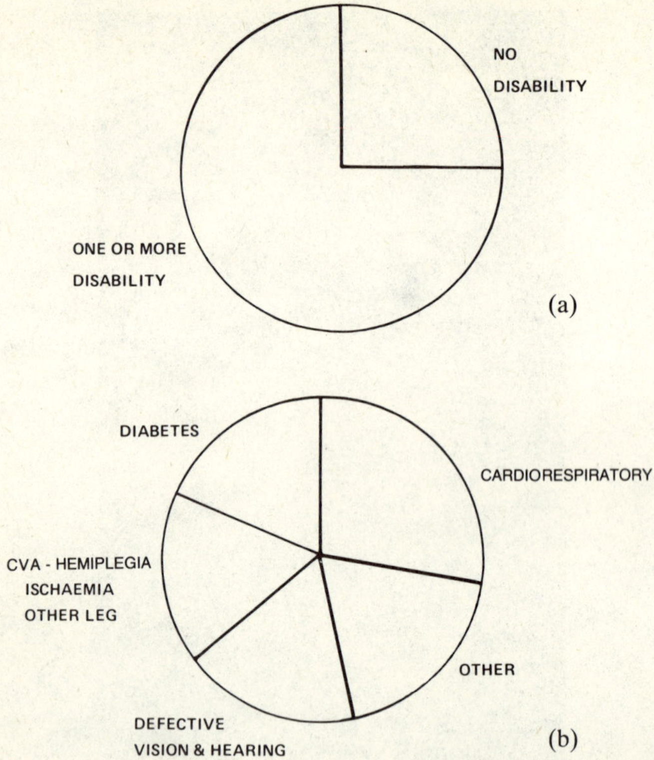


**Figure 4.2** Concurrent disabilities affecting function seen in random sample of geriatric cases

amputation, the greater is the functional loss. Thus the surgeon must consider at what level he is to operate to give viable tissues, likely to survive operation, and at the same time maximise the functional result. The constant aim should be preservation of the knee joint.

The patient within this group naturally requires a great deal of nursing care, and not only must the natural process of rehabilitation proceed but, equally, the concurrent problems require routine care and attention.

## Tumour

Tumours fortunately are rare, but it is disturbing that they do occur and are an indication for amputation in the younger age groups. The patient, often an exuberant teenager, may suffer this catastrophic happening which changes his entire way of living and almost certainly alters all his future aspirations. The cause is usually a sarcoma of the bone or soft tissue. The prognosis despite modern therapy must always be guarded. It means that surgery must be performed at rather a higher level, usually a joint intervening between the disease site and the amputation level. This ensures that amputation is done through healthy tissue. Despite the poor prognosis these patients require vigorous prosthetic management and even in the presence of metastatic spread of the disease, the doctor and nurse, with all the specialised technical aid available, cannot remain inactive in the patient's eyes.

Neoplastic change can of course be seen in the elderly patient. Epitheliomatous change can occur at the site of chronic ulceration of the lower leg and the first indication of the problem may be a pathological fracture of the tibia. This makes amputation inevitable (Figure 4.3).

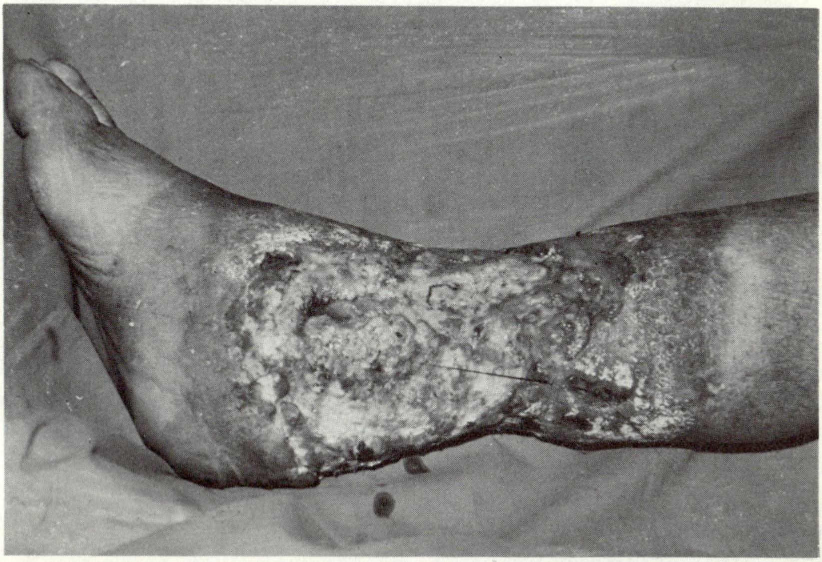

**Figure 4.3** Long standing ulceration complicated by epitheliomatous change involving bone

## Trauma or injury

Trauma or injury leading to amputation naturally affects all age groups but, generally speaking, it is seen more frequently as a result of industrial or road traffic accidents (Figure 4.4). Usually there is no question of vascular insufficiency other than that caused by the injury and the surgeon may decide on a two stage operation. His first thought is to save as much tissue as possible and then, at a later date, he will carry out a more definitive procedure.

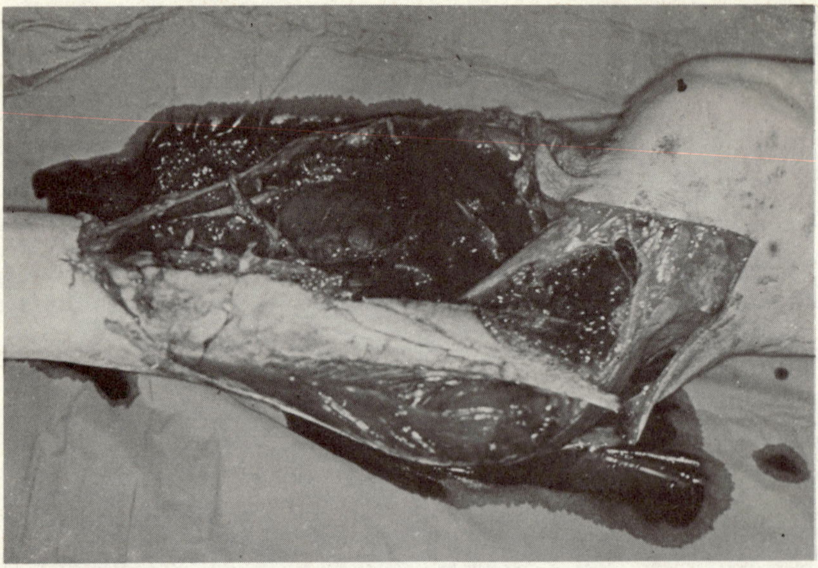

**Figure 4.4** Severe lower leg injury resulting from road traffic accident

## Chronic infection

Chronic bone infection or osteomyelitis was at one time a common disease. Antibiotics changed this in a large percentage of cases but there are still infections which do not respond even to vigorous and prolonged antibiotic therapy. This may result in such conditions as pathological fractures and discharging sinuses, causing severe inconvenience and disability. Thus amputation carried out for chronic infection tends to be accepted willingly by the few patients involved.

## Paralysis, deformity, and limb discrepancy

Paralysis, usually the result of poliomyelitis, although likely to be rare in the future, is still seen from past epidemics. In general it is accompanied by deformity and limb discrepancy (Figure 4.5(a), (b), (c)). Treatment varies according to the site and severity of the condition and it is a complex problem for both the patient and the doctor. Frequently the treatment consists of the fitting of orthoses and/or surgical footwear. Although this may result in some improvement in function, it almost always adds to the cosmetic defect which can be considerable. This is of major importance in the young patient—cosmesis being supremely important to the young woman, especially during the second decade of life, function perhaps having greater importance to the young man. It is, of course, important not to replace static disfiguration with dynamic ugliness. Thus there are many

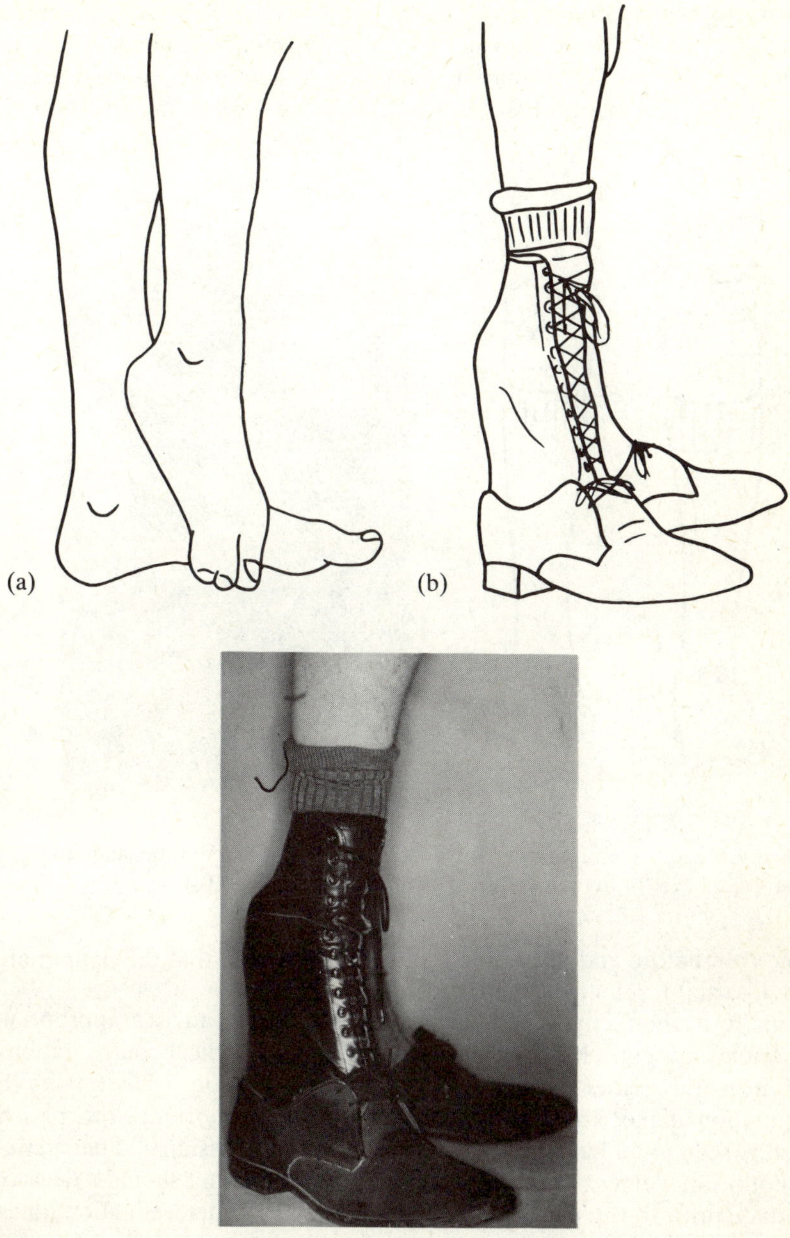


**Figure 4.5** (a) Limb discrepancy, degree shortening. (b) and (c) O'Connor extension

factors to be considered (age, sex, future aspirations, social interest, function etc.) and then, having obtained an intimate knowledge of the patient's total problem it may be necessary to advise amputation (Figure 4.6 (a) and (b)). (Note: Figures 4.5 (a)–(c) and 4.6 (a) and (b) show the

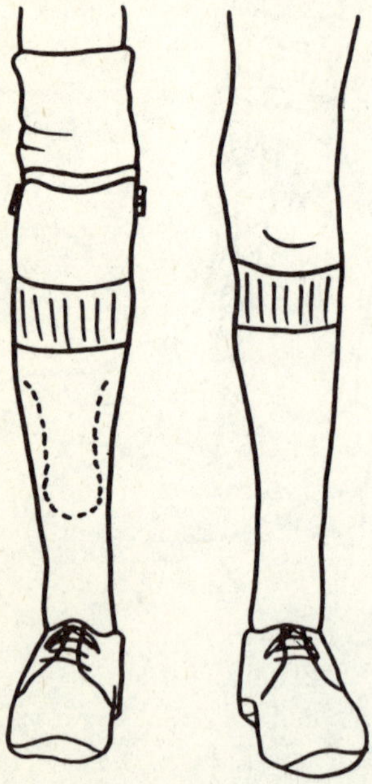

(a)

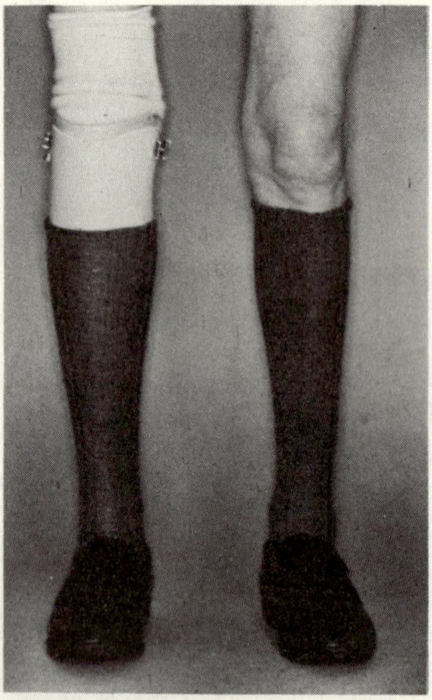

(b)

**Figure 4.6** Limb discrepancy. Conversion to Syme's amputation and fitting of prosthesis. Level of Syme's stump shown within prosthesis (a)

same case before and after operation. It will be seen that the patient also had a partial forefoot deficiency.)

Finally it should be said that the doctor simply advises appropriate treatment and gives his reason as in many other medical confrontations, and it is the patient who makes the final decision. The finality of amputation makes this confrontation extremely important—the patient must be seen to understand the implications of his decision and persuasion cannot be an element in the consultation. On no account should a decision be made prior to the patient reaching the age of self-determination unless medical necessity at an early age over-rides this situation, in which case it is the parents' decision.

## Congenital limb deficiency

Congenital limb deficiency is fortunately rare and can vary from minor deficiencies to the severe loss met in the thalidomide tragedy. Generally speaking, the latter cases are largely a prosthetic problem, perhaps with supportive orthopaedic surgical measures. The former, however, frequently involve amputation surgery. The nomenclature of congenital deficiency has been the subject of much discussion over the years and recently there

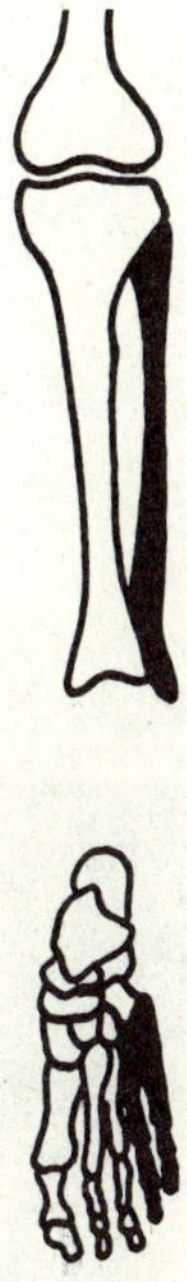

**Figure 4.7** Congenital absence of fibula

has been an attempt to agree an international code of practice. This has resulted in a classification briefly described as follows.

1 *Transverse deficiencies lower extremity*

| | |
|---|---|
| Thigh<br>Lower leg | Complete/Upper third/Middle third/Lower third |
| Tarsus<br>Metatarsus<br>Phalanges | Complete/Partial |

2 *Longitudinal deficiencies lower extremity*

| | | | |
|---|---|---|---|
| Proximal: | Femoral | (FE) | |
| Distal: | Tibial | (TI) | |
| | Central | (CE) | |
| | Fibular | (FI) | |
| | Tarsal | (TA) | Hypoplasia |
| | Metatarsal (1–5) | (MT) | Partial aplasia |
| | Phalangeal (1–5) | (PH) | |
| Combined: | Femoral | (FE) | Complete aplasia |
| | Tibial | (TI) | |
| | Fibular | (FI) | |
| | Tarsal | (TA) | |
| | Metatarsal (1–5) | (MT) | |
| | Phalangeal (1–5) | (PH) | |

The complexity of the problem remains but comprehension of nomenclature is improved.

To quote a clinical example (Figures 4.7 and 4.8) in congenital absence

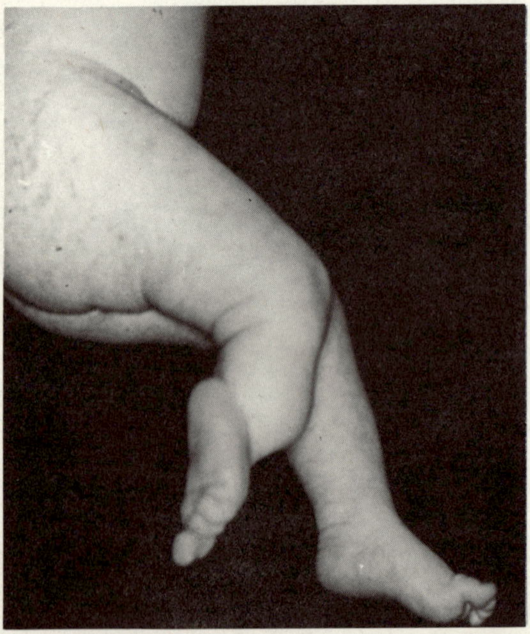

**Figure 4.8** Congenital absence of fibula

of the fibula with a severe foot deformity (combined, L or R FI/MT/PH 4/5), the common practice is ablation of the foot, with conversion to a Syme's amputation. This is by no means the ideal treatment in every case and, since it is a comparatively rare condition, it is usually dealt with by a surgeon with experience in such matters who also has a knowledge of the possible prosthetic replacement.

It will be seen that the indications for amputation are varied and that decisions involve many factors, amongst them the relative importance of function and cosmesis. It is clear that the caring team must understand and appreciate each patient as an individual and each problem as a challenge.

# 5 **Levels and Limiting Factors in Amputation Surgery**

Regardless of the level, or the presence or absence of any limiting factor, amputation surgery results in a limb stump. This may vary from minimal distal loss, e.g. the toes or partial foot, to extreme proximal loss, e.g. hindquarter. The stump, being the result of a surgical procedure largely judged for cosmetic reasons to be mutilating, is nevertheless the point of contact between the patient and the prosthesis; more accurately, the stump/socket contact point is called the interface. It is therefore seen that the stump must inevitably be responsible for the control of the prosthesis—it is in effect the 'power-house' of a new method of walking.

For these reasons the level of amputation is of extreme importance, but it is inevitably governed by limiting factors.

The common levels of amputation in the lower limb are (Figure 5.1):

1 hindquarter,
2 hip disarticulation,
3 above-knee,
4 Gritti–Stokes,
5 through-knee,
6 below-knee,
7 Syme's procedure,
8 partial foot.

Each level requires some comment since they have particular points of importance for those responsible for the patient's care.

*Hindquarter and hip disarticulation* are particularly mutilating and this may be understood when it is recognised that the cause is nearly always a tumour—usually an osteosarcoma in the region of the knee—thus the pathology determines the level. The limitation at this level is clearly the gross functional limitation imposed on the patient (Figure 5.2). Amputation at a slightly lower level, e.g. high above-knee, plus the use of modern cytotoxic drugs is now being attempted.

*Above-knee amputation* should leave as long a stump as possible to act as a good lever with adequate power to control a prosthesis. There are two important limiting factors:

1 the possible development of a hip flexion deformity following

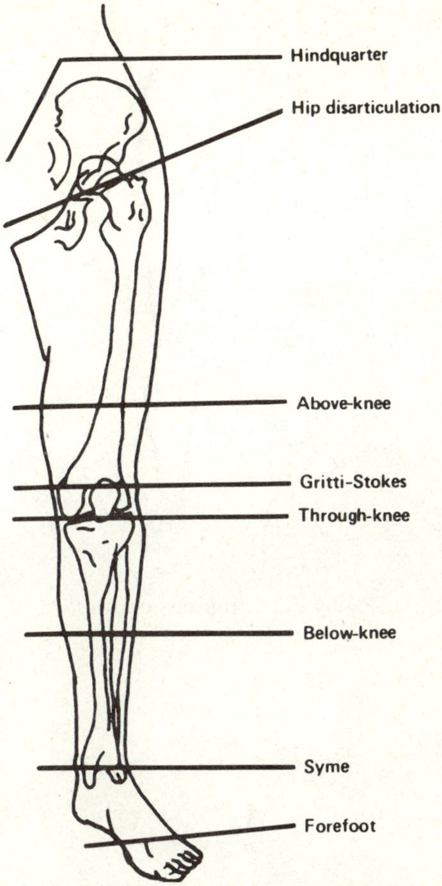


**Figure 5.1** Levels of amputation

prolonged bedrest, often associated with inadequate nursing supervision and physiotherapy. This deformity creates prosthetic problems, the socket having to be aligned in flexion (Figure 5.3). If it is present at the time of operation it may necessitate amputation at a higher level or, on the other hand, if it develops after amputation it may require a surgical release of the soft tissue at the hip.

2 the necessity to incorporate some kind of mechanical knee control in the prosthesis—this requires about 10 cm of space above the knee centre. Thus the ideal level can be said to be 10–15 cm above the knee centre in the absence of hip flexion deformity. It should be noted that some modular assembly prosthetic components do not impose this limitation.

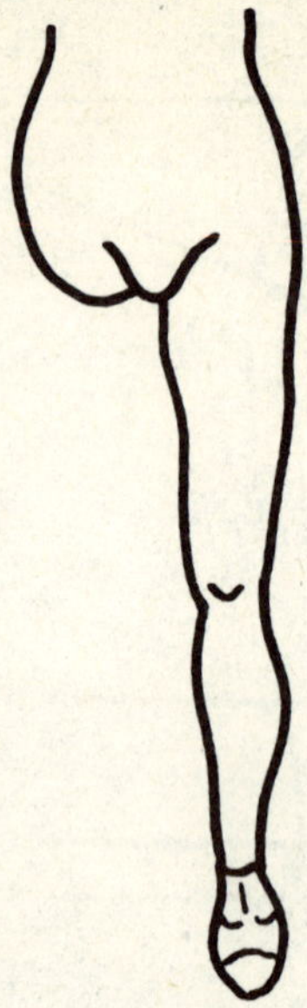

**Figure 5.2** Hip disarticulation

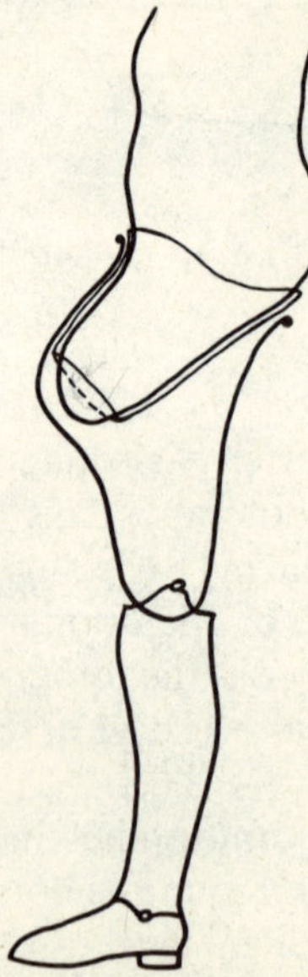

**Figure 5.3** Problem of flexed hip when fitting prosthesis results in bad cosmesis and difficult alignment

*Gritti–Stokes amputation* is an operation which should be mentioned (Figure 5.4). This is carried out at the upper level of the femoral condyles and is said to accept loading over the distal end of the stump when wearing a prosthesis. Some authorities favour this level but there is no real

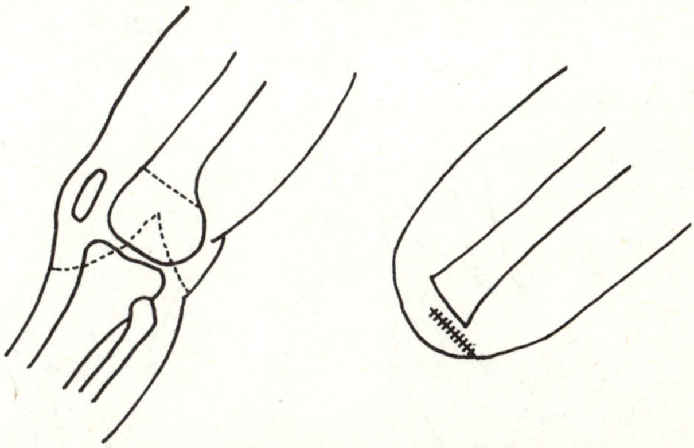

**Figure 5.4** Gritti–Stokes amputation

advantage since the final ability of the stump to bear weight is, in the authors' view, poor and end bearing tends to be unacceptable to the patient. It is also stated that amputation at this level heals readily but again, this can be disputed. Prosthetic fitting is difficult due to the proximity of the knee centre.

*Through-knee amputation* (Figure 5.5) is a useful procedure and has both advantages and limiting factors. The end of the stump in this case is,

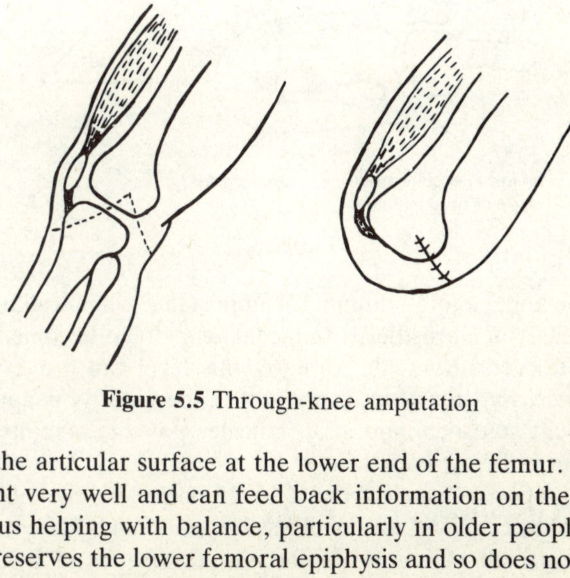

**Figure 5.5** Through-knee amputation

of course, the articular surface at the lower end of the femur. It therefore bears weight very well and can feed back information on the position of the limb thus helping with balance, particularly in older people. In young people it preserves the lower femoral epiphysis and so does not inhibit the growth potential. However, cosmesis is not good with the prostheses currently available. This is because the knee becomes bulky and, as will be seen later, it is necessary to incorporate side steels to give a knee joint. Recently four bar linkage knee units have given the facility of containing the knee joint within the limb contour but cosmesis tends to be deficient due to an excessively long thigh. A further limiting factor, as with above-knee levels, is the presence of hip flexion deformity.

*Below-knee amputation* (Figures 5.6, 5.7) is of importance since it

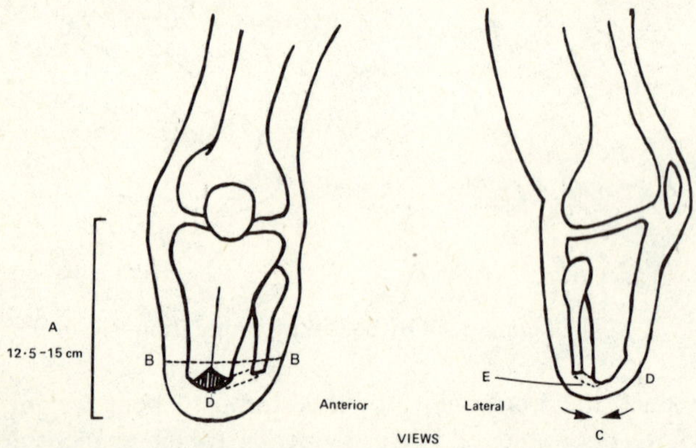


**Figure 5.6** Below-knee amputation. A, length; B, anterior scar from long posterior flap; C, opposing muscle suture; D, shaping of tibia; E, bony bridge which can be formed in the osteomyoplastic procedure

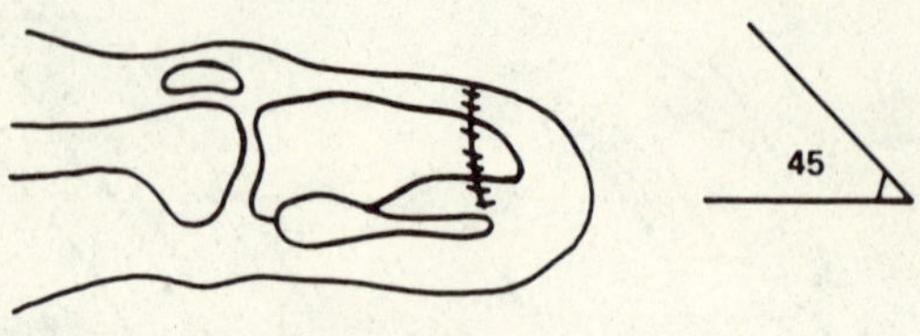


**Below-knee stump showing suture line and angle of tibial sculpting**

**Figure 5.7**

preserves the knee, a joint of immense importance when walking, especially for the wearer of a prosthesis. In recent years it has become increasingly obvious that, even in vascular disease, this level can prove viable. The benefit of increased function, especially in the elderly, is apparent. The authors' recent statistical appraisal indicates possible viability in 78% of primary cases at below-knee level.

The amputation is carried out 12.5–15 cm below the tibial plateau. Prosthetic replacement at this level has become much more sophisticated in recent years but a limiting factor is the presence of a knee flexion deformity. A further factor, which must be mentioned as such, is an apparent reluctance of surgical opinion to accept that a below-knee level may be achieved in cases presenting with vascular disease, by far the most common reason for primary amputation in Western Europe. There is little doubt that practical experience challenges this opinion and below-knee levels can, and do, prove perfectly feasible.

*Syme's procedure* (Figure 5.8) has been accepted for many years and has enormous value in that it produces a stump which can accept the full body

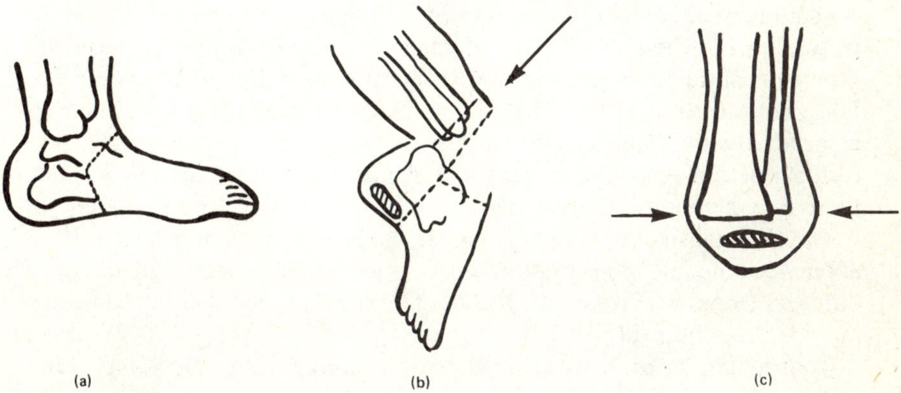


**Figure 5.8** Syme's procedure: (a) line of incision; (b) disarticulation at ankle; (c) tips of malleoli removed, heel pad in position

weight. The technique of operation uses the heel pad which is naturally designed to accept loads, but there are very obvious limiting factors. The stump end; being bulbous, does not result in a satisfactory prosthetic cosmesis around the ankle and for this reason it may be unacceptable to the female patient. If this procedure is used for limb discrepancies it may be possible, given sufficient shortening, to accommodate the bulbous end within the normal prosthetic calf contour, thereby producing an acceptable cosmesis.

A further disadvantage is the likelihood of the level being non-viable in the great proportion of cases of peripheral vascular disease, although viability may be achieved in the diabetic.

*Partial foot amputation* is carried out in many ways at varying levels. The critical consideration is the final functional result, often less than satisfactory.

Thus, it will be seen that various levels have their advantages, disadvantages, and limiting factors. It is essential that these be recognised in any preoperative assessment since failure to do so may result in discomfort, diminished function and impaired cosmesis for the amputee in the future.

# 6 Preoperative Care

As has been said amputation of a lower limb may be necessary for a variety of reasons but the majority of patients (85%) are within the geriatric age group and suffer from peripheral vascular disease with or without diabetes. Since the patient is elderly, he may in all likelihood have other handicaps associated with advancing years, e.g. cardiac failure, osteoarthritis, or a residual hemiplegia. The ischaemic foot may be infected, and in addition there may be considerable pain.

The hospital surroundings will be strange and the patient will be anxious about the outcome of his treatment. At times he will be confused and quite different from his normal self. It should be remembered that the confusion may be drug induced.

Counselling, as in many medical confrontations is extremely important. Indeed it is of greater importance in amputation surgery because the treatment clearly results in an irretrievable situation. Advice may have to be given to a parent in the case of a young child or to a family member in the case of an elderly patient who may well be confused and unable to arrive at any decision. It may be necessary to arrange for the patient to meet and talk with an established amputee of the same age and suffering from a functional loss similar to the one which will result from treatment. The use of film and video recordings can often be useful especially when dealing with parents and the disabled child. The implications of limb loss are difficult for the patient to comprehend and any counselling must, as far as possible, bear in mind the patient's fears, aspirations, and way of life.

When it has been decided that amputation is necessary, whatever the cause, the surgeon should explain to the patient and to his relatives the reasons for amputation and outline the rehabilitation programme to follow. He will obtain the patient's consent to operate and the appropriate form will be completed. During the days or weeks the patient is in hospital prior to amputation, every effort should be made to ensure that he is as fit as possible for this major operation and for his subsequent rehabilitation.

There should be a team approach to his care (Figure 6.1) that is, the surgeon, physician, nurse, and physiotherapist all have a part to play in caring for the patient, giving him reassurance and encouragement. The medical social worker and the occupational therapist may be involved. The prosthetist is mainly concerned with postoperative care but his professional skill is also of value preoperatively.

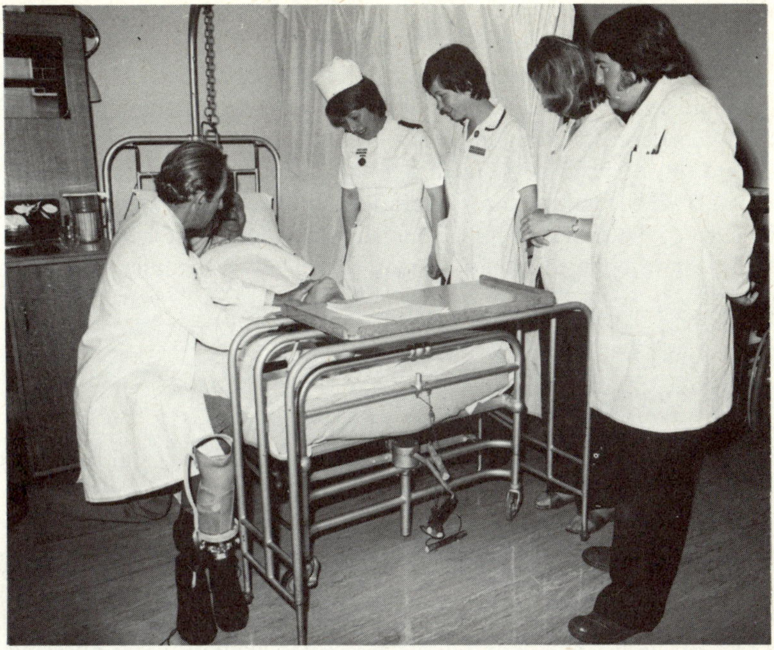

**Figure 6.1** The preoperative caring team

## Relief of pain

It is essential that analgesics be given promptly and in adequate dosage, for the pain in peripheral vascular disease may be severe and unremitting. There are two types of pain both of which may be present:

1 throbbing pain—this is thought to be pregangrenous because it is often associated with changes in the colour of the skin. This type of pain is eased if the limb is kept cool.
2 burning pain—this seems to extend from the sole of the foot and is considered to be due to ischaemic neuropathy.

Thus the patient may gain comfort by thrusting the foot outside the bedclothes and allowing it to be dependent over the side of the bed. Elevating the head of the bed on 15 cm blocks sometimes helps since this too may cause increased circulation to the feet—this is contraindicated if there is much oedema.

A bedcradle suitably placed will help by relieving the weight of the bedclothes on the feet.

A narcotic is usually necessary to ensure a good night's sleep.

## Diet

A nourishing, easily digested diet with added vitamins will help to improve the patient's general medical condition. If he is a diabetic a suitable diet should be ordered, bearing in mind that his insulin requirements may have increased during his illness. In this connection the control of the unstable diabetic, both before and after operation, may best be achieved by using a sliding scale of soluble insulin. This should be continued to the stage of mobilisation when insulin requirement is reduced and stabilisation is finally achieved.

## Care of the contralateral foot

Every effort should be made to keep the unaffected foot and leg healthy, remembering that this will soon be the patient's only foot, and that during the early stages of mobilisation it will be his main support point. In addition it may also be the site of peripheral vascular disease but to a lesser degree.

Inspect the foot carefully every day to make sure the skin on the heel and over the malleoli remains undamaged. Provided there is no abrasion or discoloration, wash the foot in warm water and dry it carefully, especially between the toes. Massage the pressure areas gently with a little surgical spirit; use olive oil if the skin is hard and dry (Figure 6.2). Use talcum powder sparingly. Treat abrasions with sterile dressings; use ribbon gauze 2.5 cm between the toes if the skin there is damaged.

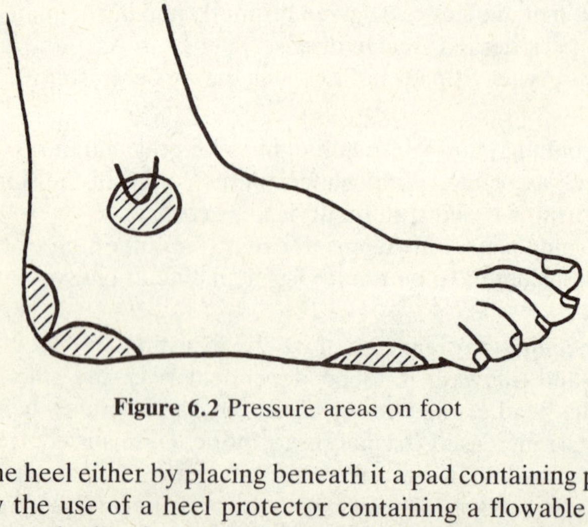

**Figure 6.2** Pressure areas on foot

Protect the heel either by placing beneath it a pad containing polystyrene beads or by the use of a heel protector containing a flowable aggregate. Both these methods of protection avoid any high loading over bony prominences and preserve the vitality of the skin. Do not use sheepskin either as a pad or muff if there is any sign of gangrene as, in the ischaemic foot, it may increase skin temperature to the extent of producing pain.

Examine the patient's shoes to make sure they are suitable for standing or walking. Their fit should be broad and long enough to avoid pressure on the toes. Avoid the use of slippers since they generally give very inadequate support.

## Control of infection

Bedrest may be necessary if there is much infection in the affected foot. Antibiotics may be ordered after bacteriological examination to determine the infecting organisms and their sensitivity, and local applications may be required. In general, antibiotics are of doubtful value in cases of peripheral vascular disease because of the inadequate tissue drug concentrations achieved due to the vascular problem. It must be remembered that heat has an adverse effect on devitalised tissue, and that soaks or wet dressings may cause maceration of the tissues.

## Medical procedures

Certain routine investigative procedures are necessary such as a chest X-ray and an electrocardiogram, recording of blood pressure, and urinalysis. Specimens of venous blood will be sent to the appropriate departments for estimation of the haemoglobin, serum electrolytes, and plasma glucose levels and for cross-matching since a transfusion may be required. Recent studies seem to indicate in peripheral amputations that increased blood viscosity can delay or even prevent healing and the question as to whether or not transfusion is necessary must be considered carefully.

Many investigative methods used to determine amputation level have been described over the years. Most are associated with an estimation of the blood flow and are not necessarily a reliable guide to a precise level. Some are of undoubted value in assessing the possibility of vascular surgery.

Aortography and femoral arteriography give indications of the status of the vascular tree. Both are of importance—the former in showing the status from the aorta down to the knee including the aortic bifurcation, often the site of massive thrombus formation and the latter in showing the status below the knee. Disobliteration of a vessel or bypass surgery may be found to be possible. However both procedures do not give a reliable indication of tissue viability in amputation surgery.

Oscillometry, a quantitative measurement of arterial pulsation obtained by using a cuff and a recording device, is of little value.

Plethysmography, a technique known for many years, relies on venous occlusion and measurement of the increase in limb volume resulting from the peripheral circulation. It is also of little value.

More recently isotope clearance methods have been used. Fairly precise figures of peripheral blood flow can be obtained but because of the technique these figures only apply to very limited areas of tissue. In addition they are invasive and are not recommended in the assessment of amputation level.

Various methods of estimation of skin blood pressure and blood flow have been described and no doubt have their individual value.

Doppler methods have also been used. They enable vessels to be detected when normal clinical methods fail and recordings of systolic blood pressure within these vessels can be made. It has been stated that these pressures, expressed as a percentage of the individual's normal brachial pressure, give a good indication of level viability. However, this method does not measure actual tissue perfusion and for this reason it is of doubtful value in estimation of level.

By far the most useful investigative procedure is thermography. It is non-invasive and gives a picture of the skin temperature variation of the whole limb. As a routine measure it is easily carried out. However, the technique must be rigidly controlled and the environment must be correct since ambient room temperature is very significant. The physicist carrying out the investigation must be highly skilled and the interpretation of the findings is all important. Given an ideal situation the amputation level can be predicted accurately in 90% of cases. This is by far the most useful investigation available in assessing amputation level (Figure 6.3).

Immediately prior to surgery, penicillin or, if a sensitivity to penicillin exists, erythromycin should be given to prevent *Clostridium welchii* infection. A change to erythromycin may also be necessary if penicillin resistant organisms are found in the affected leg prior to surgery. Parenteral administration is continued for two to three days and then the drug is given orally for a total of one week. Following surgery a five day course of miniheparin appears to help in the prevention of deep venous thrombosis.

## Preparation of limb for surgery

It is essential to check and record which limb is to be amputated. The actual skin preparation varies from hospital to hospital and from surgeon to surgeon, but it is always necessary to wash the limb and dry it carefully. Some surgeons like the first skin preparation to be done in the ward using a detergent in the washing water and then a bacteriostatic skin application, followed by drying with a sterile towel and enclosure in a sterile wrap. Others prefer to complete the skin preparation themselves in the theatre.

The method currently in use by the authors is as follows. Two days before amputation the whole limb is washed and dried. A povidone–iodine

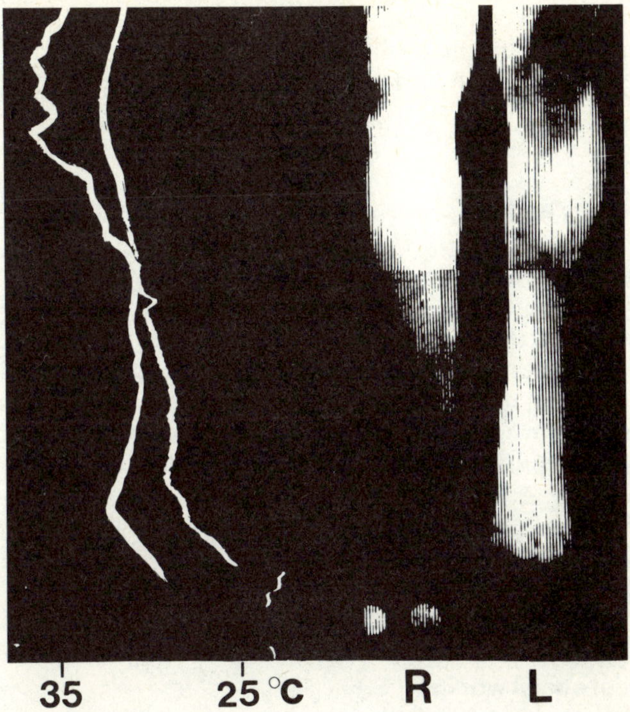


**Figure 6.3** Thermogram of the anterior aspect of the lower limbs of a patient with a severely ischaemic right foot. There is extensive hyperthermia around the right knee which is indicative of collateral circulation there. The temperature gradient on the right side falls from the below-knee level and is especially severe along the foot. A below-knee amputation is indicated

wet wrap is then applied for two hours, removed, and the limb is enclosed in sterile dry wraps. These wet and dry wraps are repeated on the following day. The wraps extend either to above the knee or to the groin, depending on the proposed level of amputation. A final povidone–iodine wet wrap is applied two hours preoperatively and left *in situ*. If the foot is infected it is enclosed in a plastic bag, the top of which is sealed to the skin, the final povidone–iodine wrap extending upwards from the sealed level.

Normally an aperient is given to the patient two evenings before operation. No food or oral liquids are given during the eight hours preceding surgery.

Prior to leaving the ward the patient empties his bladder, he is dressed in a theatre gown, and perineal drapes are applied. A theatre sock is put on his contralateral leg. Dentures are removed. Premedication is checked and given according to the anaesthetist's instructions. X-rays and case sheets with the side and probable site of amputation clearly indicated are taken with the patient to theatre.

The actual site of amputation in vascular disease can be determined only by the surgeon at the time of operation. If the skin flaps fail to bleed adequately at the proposed level it will be necessary to amputate at a higher level.

## Physiotherapy and the prevention of flexion deformities

The physiotherapist will help to prevent or correct flexion deformities of the hips and the knees with extension exercises, and she should show the nurse how to extend each hip in turn when the patient's pressure areas are being treated. The mattress should have a firm base to prevent it from sagging—a sagging mattress tends to cause hip flexion. The patient will be encouraged to move his arms and to practise deep-breathing. If he is well enough the physiotherapist will assist him to stand and, if possible, walk a little between walking rails in order to improve muscle tone and to stimulate the circulation. It is advisable that the patient be as independent as possible, therefore he should be encouraged to use his own muscles to move himself about the bed and from bed to chair.

## The medical social worker

One cannot expect the patient to relax comfortably in hospital if he has home worries. The medical social worker is a valuable member of the team caring for the amputee. She can help to solve many of the problems, either financial or social, which may face a family when a relative is undergoing major surgery. Her advice should be sought early so that she has time to make any necessary arrangements.

## Occupational therapy

If the patient is well enough to undertake any form of occupational or diversional therapy he should be encouraged to do so in order to occupy his mind and improve his general well being. Remedial therapy may be helpful since the ability to grasp with both hands will help him considerably when he begins walking training.

These arrangements might be seen as the ideal but it has to be admitted that where pain is extreme, toxicity well established, and demoralisation imminent, the patient's interests are often best served by amputation as soon as it can be arranged. In these circumstances some elements of care may have to be 'telescoped' as far as possible.

# 7 Significant Features of Amputation Surgery

It is not necessary in a publication of this type to describe in detail the surgery involved in amputation but it is essential to define certain basic principles and to mention specific points applicable to the various levels of amputation.

Surgical techniques are not only designed around the levels but are associated with the indications for the amputation. Vascular disease, trauma, deformity or discrepancy, infection and tumour all require a different type of approach. There is one common factor—the retention of tissues where considered clinically possible. This applies to soft tissue and the skeletal structure but is subject to certain functional limitations compatible with prosthetic fitting. One example of prime importance is retention of the knee in vascular disease since function is assured if this is possible; indeed it is the essence of good management of the vascular case, especially in the older age groups. In trauma there is a different approach—in a sense the level is predetermined and often the first surgical procedure is simply the removal of dead and clearly non-viable tissue. Indeed the amputation may be traumatic, limb severance occurring at the time of injury. On the other hand tissues of the limb may have been subjected to laceration and crushing which frequently involve main vessels. Later a secondary, definitive procedure can be undertaken very often using osteomyoplastic techniques. In the case of deformity or discrepancy future function must be borne in mind. There is little point in replacing deformity with reduced function. Infection and tumour demand complete eradication and there can be no doubt that positive decisions are necessary regarding the level. In all these conditions the tissues must be managed with specific aims in view—the bone may require sculpting, the muscles may require attachment to bone under tension, and the skin must be treated with great care especially in the vascular case. The tensioning of skin sutures is critical—necrosis of the wound edge can very easily be caused. Nerves and blood vessels also require special care, the former to prevent the occurrence of painful neuromata in the future.

All levels have points worthy of mention.

## Through-hip and hindquarter

These operations are considered together since a through-hip may often develop, as surgery is undertaken, into a hindquarter. The diagnosis around the hip can easily be less certain inasmuch as tumour invasion, and this is the normal cause for such a procedure, is difficult to ascertain. There are three main tumours affecting the lower limb:

1 osteosarcoma,
2 chondrosarcoma,
3 osteoclastoma.

### Osteosarcoma

Many of these may have been treated by irradiation prior to presenting for surgery. There is doubt as to whether irradiation, amputation, or both should be the treatment of choice. One thing is certain—a tumour in the region of the distal femur demands high amputation—through-hip in most cases. At the proximal end of the femur it may be possible to carry out a hindquarter but if the tumour invasion is extensive and cannot be completely excised, irradiation may be the treatment of choice. If excision is attempted and only partly achieved the final result will be a fungating wound with massive spread of tumour—the final prognosis is the same but the terminal illness is much worse.

### Chondrosarcoma

Efficacy of irradiation and the extent of surgery is again in doubt. In some cases local excision of a low grade tumour is possible, but in many, amputation at an adequate level is necessary. Very occasionally an internal prosthesis is said to be of value, e.g. replacement of the proximal half of the femur.

### Osteoclastoma

Curettage of this type of tumour is undertaken initially in order to establish the diagnosis. In some cases a cure results but in many there must be a decision at a later date between irradiation and amputation or excision. Again an internal prosthesis may be of value.

Preoperative assessment must include biopsy and also the local extent of the tumour must be determined. It is a severe surgical procedure involving considerable blood loss and demanding quite specifically, specialised surgery.

## Above-knee

Indications are more numerous at this level. Consideration of the final stump function must govern the amputation technique. The stump itself must be so fashioned as to allow the wearing of a prosthesis—there must also be control. In no way can the sectioned end of the femur accept weight bearing. The surface area is small and the skin flap covering the bone, along with muscle, would not survive. Mid-thigh amputation divides the thigh adductors and extensors and these may be anchored to bone in order to allow the hip to function. There are several ways in which the stump can be made powerful and capable of prosthetic control. The opposing muscle groups (extensors/flexors, abductors/adductors) can be sutured together and to bone. All the muscle groups can be individually sutured to bone. Finally the adductor and hamstrings can be sutured to bone and the anterior group can be brought over to the posterior group in order to cover the bone end. In all these procedures the muscles must be tensioned correctly in order to allow them to function and, after trimming to the correct length, they can be divided. In vascular cases the surgical interference is kept to a minimum and perhaps the main object of muscle suture is covering of the sectioned femoral end.

The medulla of the sectioned bone should be closed in order to maintain intramedullary pressure. This has a distinct bearing on the structure and strength of the bone and is generally achieved by using periosteal flaps.

Exsanguination of the limb is achieved prior to surgery by using an Esmarch bandage—considerable blood loss can be avoided by this procedure.

Nerve division, as in all amputations, is important. It is carried out with the nerve under tension in order that the sectioned end retracts into the remaining muscle bulk, thereby protecting the inevitable neuroma and limiting the possibility of pain in the stump at a later date.

Finally, adequate drainage must be assured by the use of vacuum drainage. Haematoma formation is minimised by this procedure.

## Through-knee

This surgical procedure is less common—this is perhaps because of the relatively poor final prosthetic cosmesis or there may be other technical problems associated with the level. It is not a popular surgical event and delayed healing can be seen—this can be due to the underestimation of the amount of skin flap required to close the wound.

It is a relatively simple procedure, being purely a disarticulation. There is no damage to bone or cartilage and only minimal muscle section. The patella is left *in situ* and the patellar tendon, after removal from the tibial tubercle, is sutured to the cruciate ligaments. The resulting stump is strong, accepting end bearing without any problem. In children there is retention of the lower femoral epiphysis.

## Below-knee

This level is by far the commonest seen in the lower limb. Biomechanically it is acceptable since there is only a single joint loss. The prosthetic potential is wide and although the ideal stump can be defined, variations in several parameters can be successfully fitted. The optimum level of below-knee amputation involves only one relevant muscle section—the gastrocnemius—even this can be utilised to obtain improved stump function and knee control. The bony section is normally 12.5–15 cm below the knee centre and in children it may be necessary to retain as long a stump as possible even including the lower tibial epiphysis. Bone section must be carefully carried out with rounding or sculpting of the anterior contour to avoid sharp bony prominences which would cause problems with prosthetic fitting. In the younger person the sectioned ends of the tibia and fibula are joined by a periostial tube which promotes the growth of a bony bridge. The advantage of this is that the stump obtains a rigid skeletal structure, making it inherently stronger when controlling and accepting a prosthesis.

Normally the skin flaps are fashioned to give a long posterior flap and an anterior transverse scar. The long posterior flap tends to be less ischaemic and healing is more likely.

In vascular cases the aim is careful handling of tissues, minimal surgical trauma and very meticulous skin suturing. Rarely is it wise to proceed to the osteomyoplasty with the tibiofibular bony bridge and the tightly tensioned muscle flaps.

## Syme's

This procedure has stood the test of time and there have been few modifications since it was introduced by James Syme of Edinburgh in 1842. It is generally carried out for trauma, foot deformity, trophic ulceration, or limb discrepancy. In vascular disease it is infrequently used although in small vessel disease associated with diabetes it can provide a viable stump.

The surgery involves disarticulation at the ankle with removal of the malleoli and the tibial articular surface, leaving a weight bearing bony area which is at right angles to the load line in the sagittal and coronal planes. The incision allows the heel pad to be retained—this is highly significant since the tissues in the pad have the ability to withstand pressure.

There are several critical features of the surgical procedure.

1 Inadequate fixation of the heel pad allows partial subluxation and

problems with future end bearing. Steinmann's pins can be used to fix the heel pad to the tibia at the time of surgery, being removed after seven to ten days.

2 An excessively narrow neck in the fashioning of the heel flap can prejudice the viability of the tissues.
3 Infection is frequently present and it is difficult to be certain surgery is adequately clear of the affected area.
4 The postoperative environment must be optimised and this can only be achieved by the use of rigid dressings.

## Partial foot

There are many and varied procedures which have been undertaken with some degree of success.

1 Chopart amputation is infrequently carried out and probably is necessitated by trauma. It consists of a disarticulation at the talus, calcaneus/navicular, cuboid level. There is a danger of stump equinus developing due to the action of the tendoachilles, and distally callosity formation is common. Adequate fixation of the opposing muscles (e.g. tibialis anterior into the neck of the talus) may prevent the former and good prosthetic fitting the latter.
2 Lisfranc is also rarely seen. The indications are similar to a Chopart. The disarticulation is at the tarsometatarsal level.
3 Trans-metatarsal amputation varies in precise level but is usually just proximal to the metatarsal heads. An adequate plantar flap is essential since the dorsal skin is not suitable for stump end cover. It is applicable in trauma and in certain cases of vascular disease, perhaps being seen as an alternative to toe amputation which frequently can fail.
4 Amputation of the toes is fairly common practice. In vascular cases the outcome is frequently in doubt and there can be nothing more demoralising for the patient than to have multiple minor amputations all of which fail, finally leading to a higher level of amputation which might have been indicated in the first instance.

It is clear that precise surgical indications exist and basic criteria must be satisfied. There is one further consideration and that is the compatibility of the procedure with prosthetic fitting. For this reason it is obvious that the surgeon must be aware of basic bioengineering principles and the possible prosthetic management in the future. If this is not so, patient care is less than adequate and the final functional results may be poor. The aim of limb ablation must be maximum replacement of function.

# 8 Postoperative Care

## The nursing and rehabilitation area

Until residential limb fitting centres are established throughout the country it will continue to be necessary to nurse the amputee either in the general wards or in special units in general hospitals. In a specialised residential centre the amputee would no longer be the 'odd man out' for he would be with a group of people, all amputees, and together with them he would look forward to living independently again.

He would have a team of people caring for him (Figure 8.1). They would

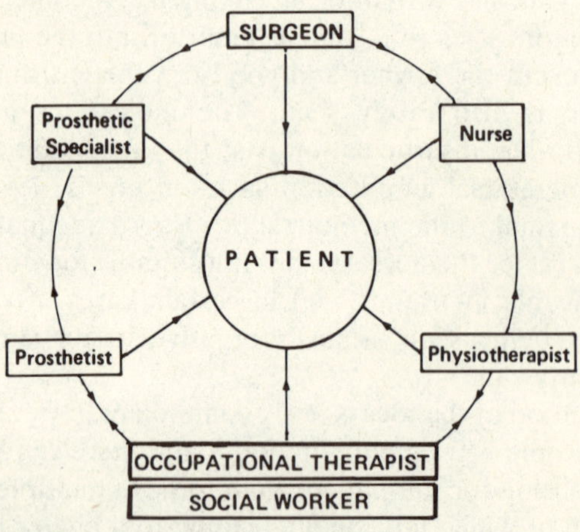


**Figure 8.1** The postoperative caring team

be members of various disciplines which when linked together would provide the 'total' care to which he is entitled. The team comprises the amputating surgeon who has considerable knowledge of prosthetic replacement, the rehabilitation specialist, the prosthetist, the nurse, the physiotherapist, the occupational therapist. The bioengineer and medical social worker may not attend the ward rounds but they are available whenever a need arises for their expertise.

The pace in such a unit must of necessity be unhurried, for the amputee is usually elderly. The atmosphere should be cheerful and encouraging; praise should be given as progress is made.

## General requirements of postoperative care

Rest periods are essential, the patient being allowed to sleep or rest on top of his bed for part of the afternoon. This is far better than sitting in a chair

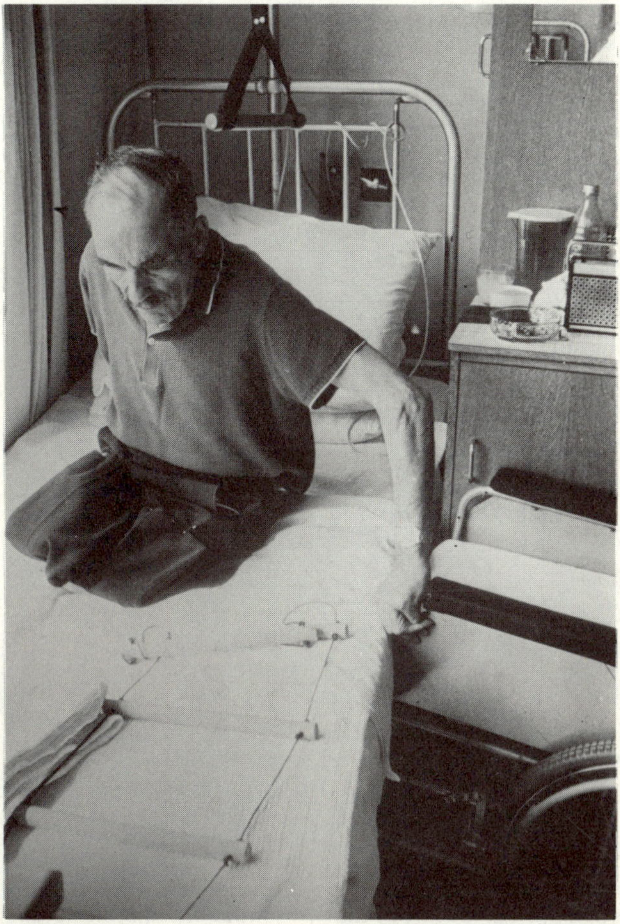

**Figure 8.2** Bed to chair transfer: overhead frame and grab handle, rope ladder

for long periods of the day as might happen with the elderly patient during which time dependency oedema may form in the remaining foot and the danger of flexion contractures may be increased.

In the care of the younger amputee the treatment offered must be much

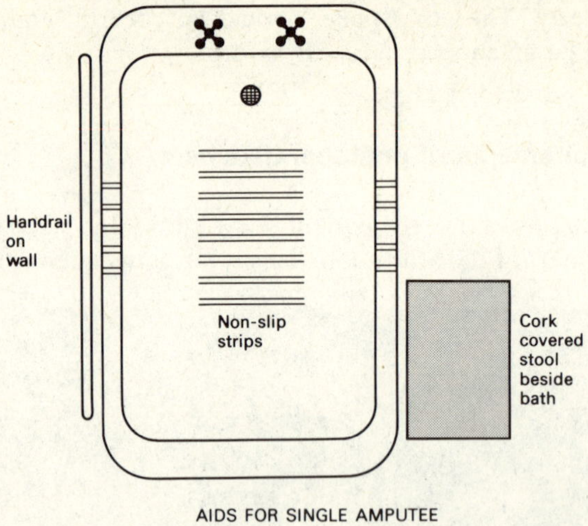


(a)

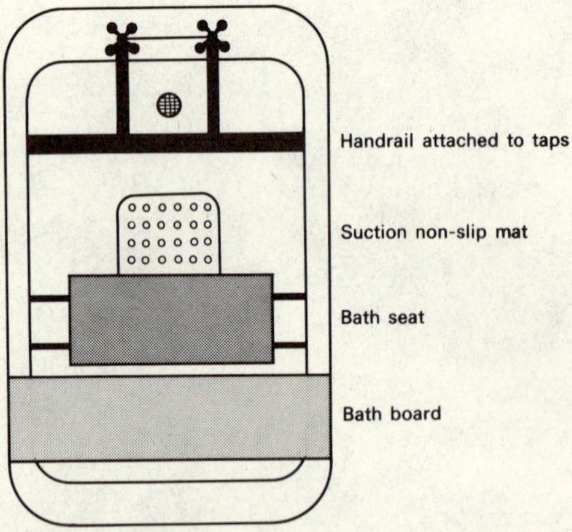


(b)

**Figure 8.3** (a)–(e) Bathing aids

more active. There is no doubt that with adequate planning this age group can be accommodated in the same unit as the older person. Treatment must vary and facilities must be present in order to offer suitable levels of activity. Although in some countries special rehabilitation units are set up for the young amputee, there may be some virtue in bringing the ages together. In addition to therapy this type of patient will need special care designed around his or her future employment and this must be an early consideration in postoperative care.

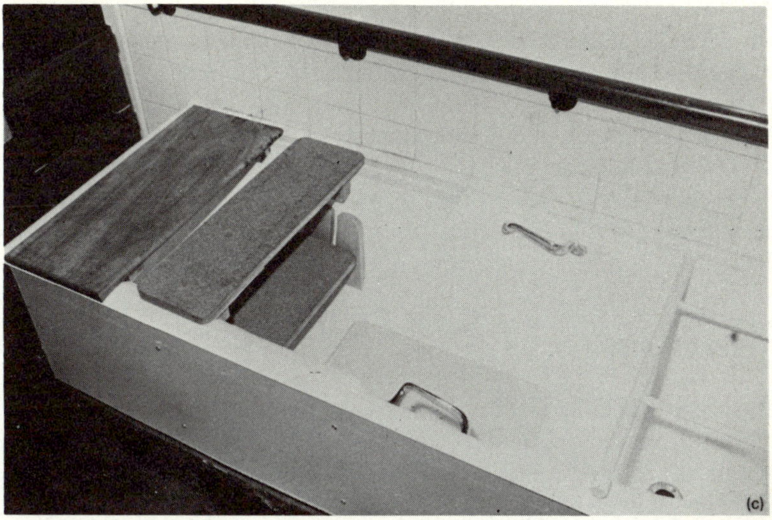


(c)

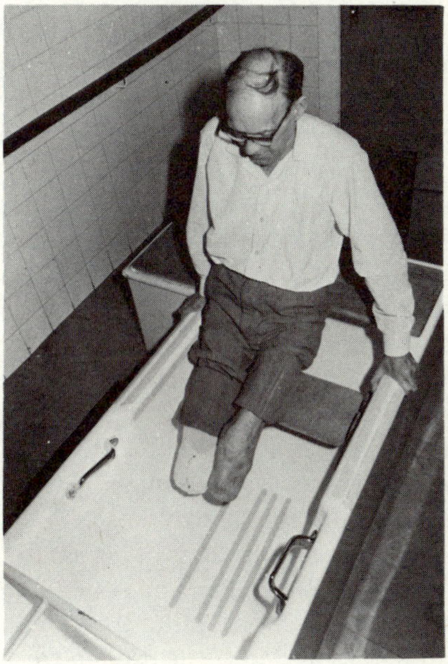

(d)

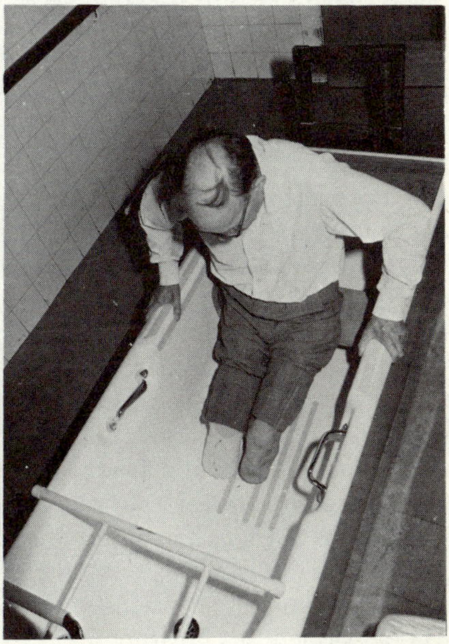

(e)

There should be sufficient space between the beds to manoeuvre the wheelchair required during the early postoperative period. Bedside lockers should be large enough to hold both day clothes and the artificial limb.

A double amputee will require a low bed, a grab handle attached to an overhead frame to grip for safety since he will now be top-heavy, and a rope ladder attached to the foot of the bed will help him to move more easily. The level of the mattress should be the same as that of the wheelchair seating to assist bed to chair transfer (Figure 8.2). A bath board and bath seat will enable him to enter and leave the bath (Figure 8.3(a)–(e)). He will need double hand-grips to assist him to transfer onto and off the toilet seat.

Wherever the amputee is nursed, the principles of nursing care are the same. However, it is preferable to care for the patient in a unit designed especially to permit a programme of total rehabilitation.

## Nursing the amputee

A freshly prepared bed with a firm base will be ready for the amputee on his return from theatre, and a bedcradle and drip-stand to hand, also a clip ready to attach the drainage bottle to the bedstead.

Lift the patient carefully on to the bed, and place him in a lateral position, his head resting on one pillow. If intravenous fluids are being given check that the apparatus is working properly.

Very often the operation site is drained through a polythene tube into a sterile vacuum bottle. Check that there is no drag on the tube, that it is not kinked, and note the amount of drainage already present. See that the antennae of the vacuum bottle are wide apart, indicating a negative pressure.

Record the patient's pulse and respiration rates every fifteen minutes and confirm that his colour is satisfactory. Record the blood pressure half-hourly and the temperature four-hourly.

Inspect the stump dressing frequently in case of unexpected haemorrhage; the stump should rest flat on the bed.

If the operation was performed under spinal anaesthesia turn the patient two-hourly to ease the pressure over bony prominences and to minimise respiratory complications. Lift the patient into a more comfortable position after twelve hours. If a general anaesthetic was used lift the patient into the semirecumbent position once he is fully conscious.

Give sips of water and mouth washes to relieve the dryness of his mouth. Drugs for the relief of pain should have been prescribed and must be given at regular intervals according to the doctor's instructions. Later the patient will be washed, his pressure areas treated, and he will be dressed in fresh clothing.

## General care

Amputation of a limb is a major operation and it is irreversible. It alters completely the patient's visual image of himself.

In many cases although the patient can see that the limb has been amputated he has the peculiar sensation that his limb is still present. This sensation known as the 'phantom limb' is quite normal and the amputee must be assured that gradually the feeling will diminish.

Occasionally both above-knee and below-knee amputees have the problem of stump tremor. This may be partly due to surgical interference with the neuromuscular mechanisms. It is most frequently manifested in the anxious patient. Reassurance and, later, firm handling of the stump by both the staff and the patient tend to alleviate the problem.

Initially the stump will be extremely tender and it must be handled gently. Pain must be relieved promptly and adequately. During the first thirty-six hours after operation a narcotic analgesic will be required at six-hourly intervals; later less addictive analgesics may be sufficient. As a rule a sedative will be required at night. All complaints of pain must be reported, since persistent pain in the early postoperative phase may indicate a problem at the operation site.

Accurate recording of the temperature, pulse, and respiration rates four-hourly is essential, as a rise in the levels accompanied by persistent pain may necessitate inspection of the wound.

Good general nursing care, including changing the patient's position frequently, will ensure comfort and avoid pressure sores since skin damage can occur remarkably quickly in cases of peripheral vascular disease.

The patient's diet should be nourishing and he should have adequate fluids.

The remaining foot should receive special care. It should be washed and dried carefully and the heel massaged gently to stimulate the circulation. If the foot feels cold a bed sock may be worn—hot water bottles are contraindicated for patients with peripheral vascular disease or diabetes mellitus. At a later stage treatment may be necessary by a chiropodist. Oedema of the foot and leg due to dependency can be controlled with a length of tubular elasticated knitted cotton of suitable size reaching from the base of the toes to the knee. In certain cases it may be necessary to prescribe an elasticated stocking.

It is most important that the patient receives 'total' care. In all probability he will require treatment for at least one of the conditions associated with old age or with atherosclerosis.

Since diabetes mellitus is a frequent cause of amputation by virtue of its associated vascular disease, treatment must be carefully supervised, bearing in mind the varying demands made by increasing activity. Opportunities must be found to make sure the patient understands the instructions on his diet sheet, and also his insulin dose.

Visual and hearing loss create a communication barrier, and so should be treated and the necessary aids supplied.

As soon as his physical condition permits the patient will be encouraged towards personal independence, to wash at the wash-basin, to dress himself, and to become independent of aid when bathing.

The double amputee will be taught it is easier for him to transfer straight forward from his wheelchair onto the toilet. He will be warned that he is top-heavy and must take care when leaning forwards to avoid falling.

If the patient's relatives have a car they should be encouraged to take him out, he will then be taught how to enter and leave the car safely. He should be encouraged to spend a weekend at home before his final discharge from the unit so that any difficulties he encounters may be discussed and remedied.

In some cases it is necessary to teach the relatives how to bandage the patient's stump and how to assist him to put on his prosthesis. It is important to reassure the relatives and to let them see for themselves the progress being made.

## Postoperative complications

### Chest infection

This is a common complication in the elderly after major surgery. Good nursing care, antibiotic cover, breathing exercises pre- and postoperatively, and the use of spinal anaesthesia help to reduce the incidence.

### Confusional state

There are many causes for this such as the strangeness of surroundings, the anaesthetic, major surgery, pain, and sleeplessness, and the use of possibly a multiplicity of analgesics. Other causes such as toxaemia, chest or renal infections may be present.

### Deep venous thrombosis and pulmonary embolism

The very nature of vascular disease predisposes towards embolic disasters. Early mobilisation, physiotherapy, and the use of miniheparin during the first five postoperative days reduce the incidence of such occurrences.

### Pressure sores

The tissues in vascular disease are very vulnerable, especially those of the contralateral foot. Careful patient assessment, the use of various aids, skilled nursing technique, and early mobilisation are essential as preventive measures (Figures 8.4 and 8.5).

### Haematoma

As the blood pressure rises postoperatively oozing may occur from a tiny blood vessel. If the wound drainage is inadequate a haematoma will form, and may cause pressure and devitalisation of the terminal tissues.

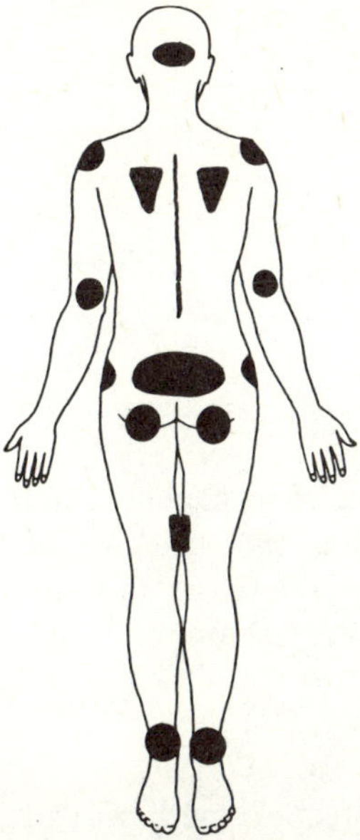

**Figure 8.4** Pressure areas on body

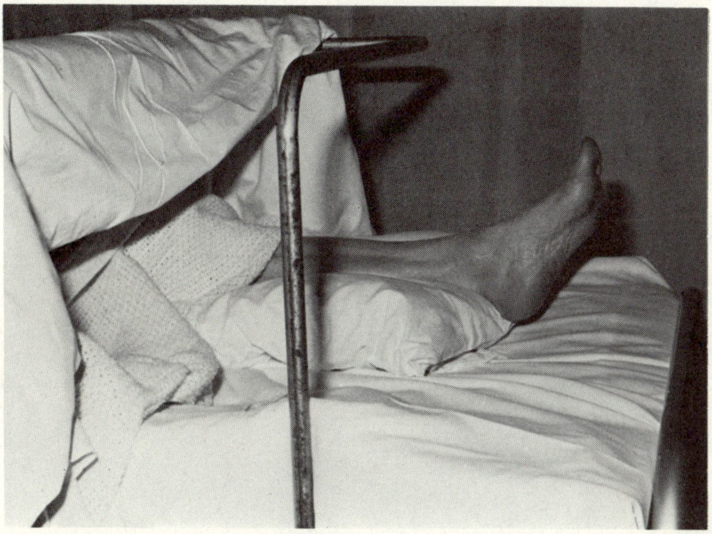

**Figure 8.5** Nursing aids

**Wound infection**

This may have been introduced at the time of injury, e.g. from a road traffic accident, or it may have been present in the ischaemic or gangrenous tissues of the amputated leg. Careful preparation of the limb for surgery and the use of antibiotic cover reduce the risk of infection.

**Wound breakdown**

Although every effort is made to choose the correct level for amputation, and to use a long posterior flap in below-knee amputations, necrosis of the skin edges may still occur, necessitating, in some cases, a wedge resection at approximately the same general level, or even revision to a higher level. Ischaemia is the common cause of wound breakdown, but infection may play a part.

**Adherent scar**

Perhaps as a result of infection or haematoma the skin may become firmly attached to the bone end so that traction on the scar occurs when the prosthesis is worn. The use of a nylon undersock (Rem–Daw sheath) may prove beneficial, but often refashioning of the stump is required.

**Sequestrum formation**

In the case of persisting infection, perhaps with a sinus, X-ray may reveal bony involvement with the possibility of sequestrum formation later.

Clearly there are other complications as seen in any surgery, particularly associated with the elderly: urinary tract infection, cardiac complications, etc.

The question of stump pain is more fully mentioned in Chapter 10.

# 9 **Stump Dressings**

The purpose of a dressing is to provide a cover for the wound in order to keep it as sterile as possible and afford it protection. Thus a dressing imposes a physical envivonment on the wound—in addition to affording sterility it creates abnormal pressures and temperatures. This has a bearing on the healing of the tissues and is an important part of amputee care.

There are several types of wound dressing:

1 simple sealing of wound using plastic sealants;
2 bandaging using crêpe bandages;
3 rigid plaster dressings
  (a) without mobility,
  (b) with mobility;
4 controlled environment treatment.

## Simple sealing of wound

This is not advised in amputation surgery because the lack of any support allows excessive post-surgical oedema to develop.

## Bandaging using crêpe bandages

On completion of the operation a non-adherent dressing is placed over the wound. This is covered with several gauze swabs. A length of sterile tube gauze is used to hold these dressings in place. The stump is then bandaged carefully but firmly in such a manner as to limit the formation of oedema at the stump end. Since a stump bandage soon becomes slack it is essential to renew it at frequent intervals without removing the inner dressings. Soft dressings are usually applied to the above-knee stump, but where they are used below the knee it is important to remember that a bandage applied too tightly may cause devitalisation of the thin skin covering the shaft of the tibia. Elasticated adhesive plaster may be used in certain circumstances and in the above-knee stump strips of this type of wound covering applied longitudinally can be effective. It must be emphasised that the tension with which they are applied is extremely important since excessive pressure can be harmful. Further, circumferential turns of such a dressing can constrict the distal stump and should never be used (see 'The healed stump' page 70).

Generally soft dressings are limited in their use to the hindquarter, through-hip, and above-knee level. They are not recommended for through-knee, below-knee, and Syme's levels. In through-knee levels the skeletal structure is very superficial and damage can easily be caused to the skin by soft dressings exerting excessive and variable pressure on the underlying bony structure. In Syme's level there is a well defined danger of subluxation of the heel pad with the use of soft dressings. This is highly significant at a later stage when the prosthesis is being fitted.

Partial foot levels are usually protected by soft dressings. The variety of surgical procedures does not allow a detailed description of the bandaging techniques. However, regardless of the extent of the amputation and particularly because of the peripheral nature any bandaging must avoid excessive localised pressure especially over any bony prominence.

**Nursing care of a patient with a soft dressing—features of importance**

1 As long as the dressings are comfortable leave them undisturbed in order to avoid introducing infection into the wound.
2 Renew the bandage every four hours. Handle the stump carefully as it will be tender.
3 Report complaints of pain so that they can be investigated and suitable treatment prescribed.
4 Provided the wound is satisfactory remove alternate sutures on the tenth day from an above-knee wound, and the remainder a few days later. As a rule allow three weeks to elapse before removing the sutures from a below-knee wound in order to ensure firm healing.
5 After removal of the sutures redress the wound with sterile gauze swabs, and renew the bandage four-hourly to maintain adequate pressure on the stump.

## Rigid plaster dressings

### Without mobility

*Hindquarter/through hip-levels*
Rigid dressings are rarely used. No advantage can be defined. There is a constant problem with suspension.

*Above-knee level*
Rigid dressings have been advocated but suspension of the dressing and maintaining contact with the wound and stump is difficult. Oedema tends to develop if this does not happen and delayed healing may result.

*Through-knee level* (Figure 9.1)
A rigid dressing is an ideal environment but care in its application is essential. Teased out swabs are applied to the distal end of the stump including the posterior aspect of the femoral condyles. A Spandex sock is

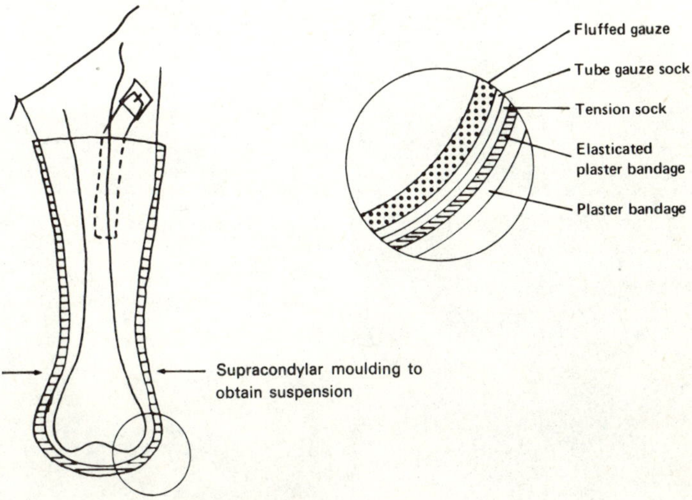


**Figure 9.1** Rigid plaster dressing, through-knee

then firmly rolled over the distal end and drawn taut at the groin. An elasticated plaster of Paris bandage followed by two rolls of ordinary plaster of Paris complete the dressing. Moulding of the plaster above the femoral condyles whilst the tautness of the Spandex sock is eased, ensures good suspension and this is reinforced by a webbing strap extending from the proximal end of the plaster to a waist belt.

*Below-knee level* (Figure 9.2 (a)–(g))
A non-adherent dressing is applied over the suture line and a few teased out gauze swabs are placed over the distal stump (Figure 9.2(a)). A specially shaped polyurethane stump end-cap may be applied instead. Both these measures ensure minimal localised pressure. Finally, a rolled sterile stump sock (Spandex) is eased over these dressings, unrolled and pulled taut (Figure 9.2(b)). The patella is protected by a shaped piece of orthopaedic felt applied on top of the sock (Figure 9.2(c)). An elasticated plaster of Paris bandage is applied and at the same time tension is maintained on the sock (Figure 9.2(d)). Ordinary plaster of Paris bandages are then applied to mid thigh (Figure 9.2(e)). The cast is carefully moulded to obtain suspension above the femoral condyles and a strap and waist-band are attached for added suspension (Figure 9.2(f)). The whole procedure is shown diagrammatically in Figure 9.2(g).

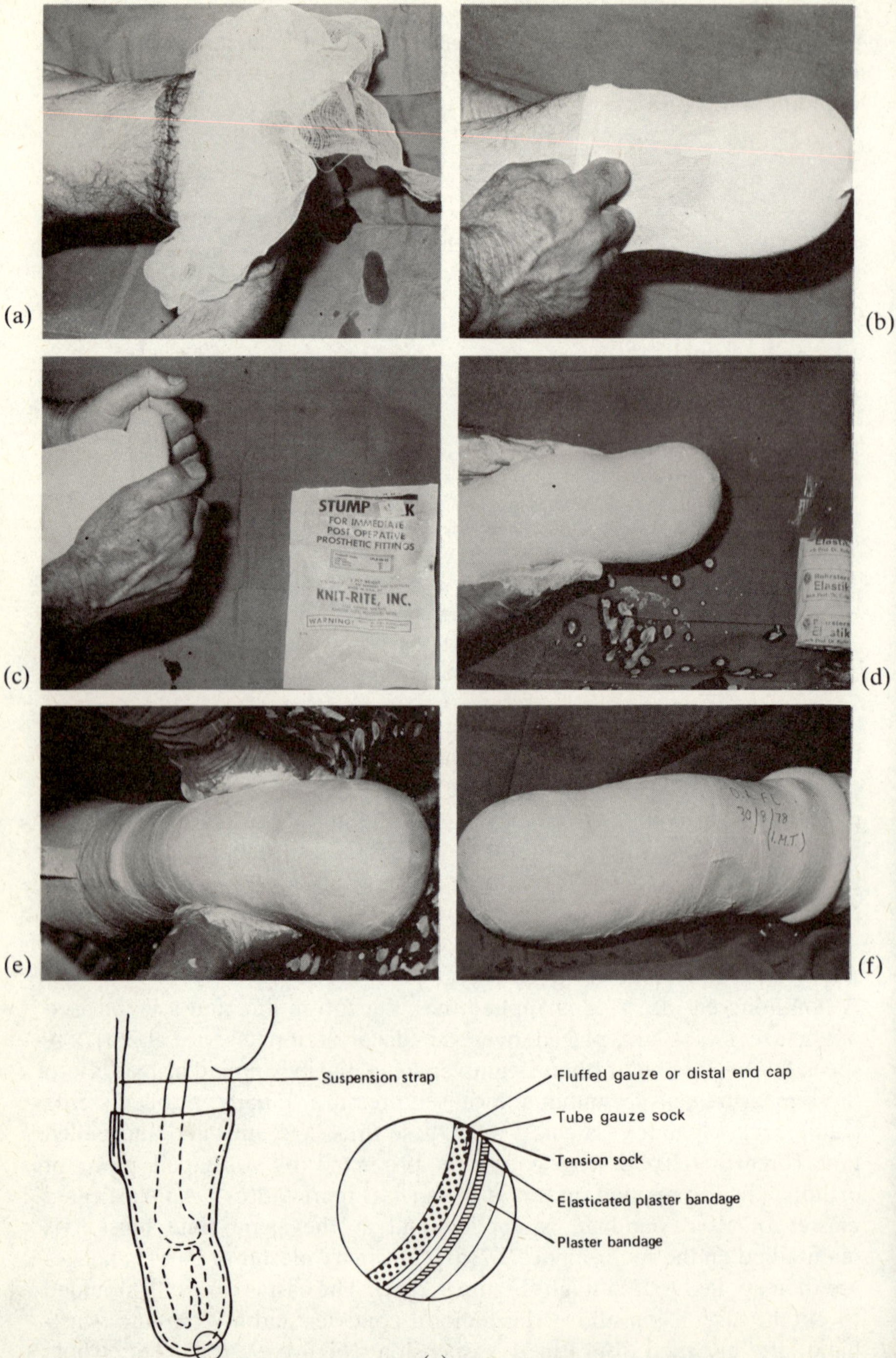


**Figure 9.2** (a)–(g) Method of application of rigid plaster dressing, below-knee

*Syme's level* (Figure 9.3)

Application is very similar at this level although it may be necessary to use a sterile shaped knitted Syme's sock instead of a Spandex. No suspension

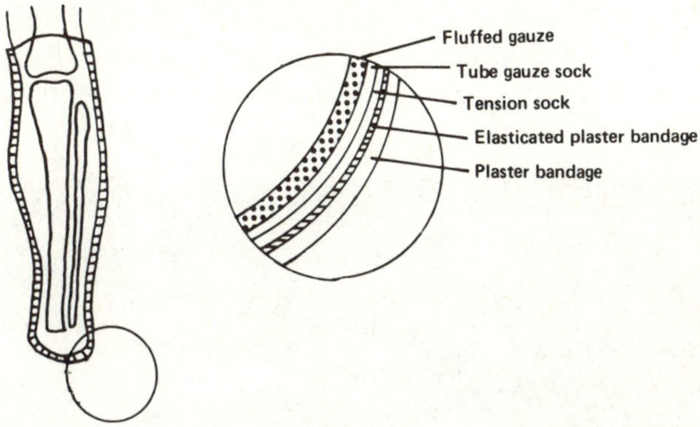


**Figure 9.3** Rigid plaster dressing, Syme's

strap is necessary, the shaping of the bulbous end of the stump being very effective in maintaining the stump/dressing relationship. The shaping of the proximal end of the rigid dressing around the tibial flare is essential in providing rotational stability between the stump and the dressing.

**With mobility** (Figure 9.4)

This is commonly known as the immediate postoperative fitting (IPOF) type plaster and is similar to the normal rigid plaster dressing without

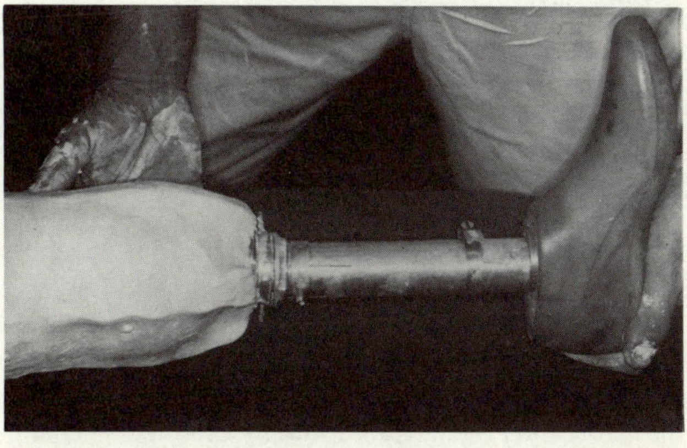

**Figure 9.4** Rigid plaster dressing with extension tube and foot, below-knee level

mobility apart from the possible addition, when used at below-knee level, of shaped orthopaedic felt. An extension tube and a prosthetic foot may be added. This enables mobilisation in the very early postoperative period, within a few days in suitable cases. It is also useful where there is delayed healing at a later stage.

Although immediate fitting techniques were used some years ago in below-knee cases allowing mobilisation on the second or third postoperative day, there is now a tendency to delay this procedure. It may even be avoided in favour of simple rigid dressings along with other means of early mobilisation. There are two exceptions—the through-knee (Figure 9.5)

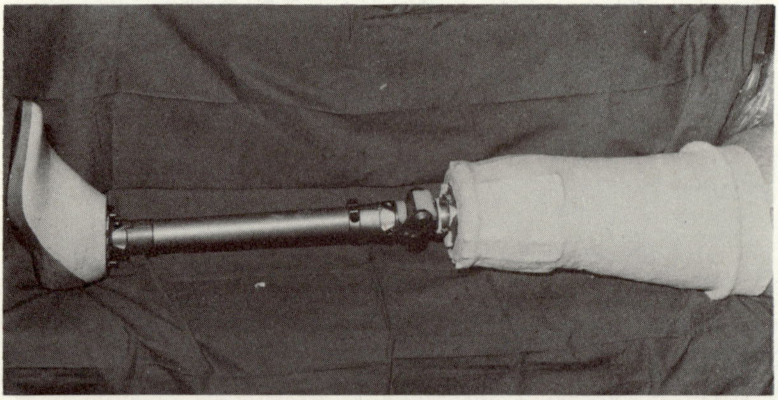

(a)

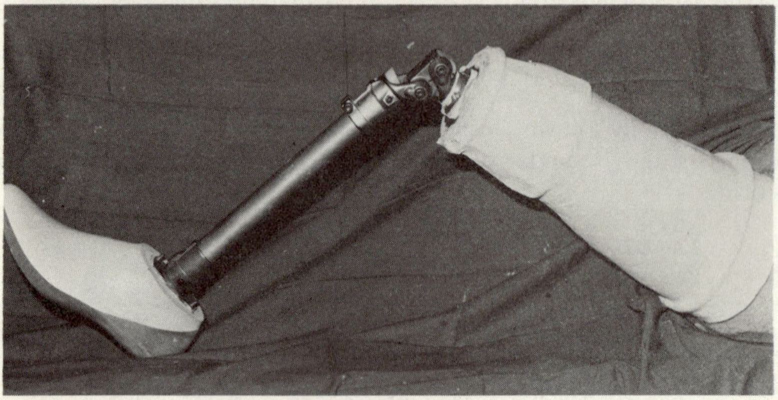

(b)

**Figure 9.5** (a) and (b) Rigid plaster dressing with extension tube and foot, through-knee level

and Syme's (Figure 9.6) levels if treated initially by rigid dressings are ideally suited to IPOF techniques at about the seventh postoperative day when the initial dressing is changed. Mobility can then be commenced and continued through the casting and fitting stages of prosthetic fabrication until final delivery. Extension tubes with alignment devices are required at all levels other than Syme's level where a Chinese rocker probably with a cork raise will suffice. A prosthetic foot is difficult to incorporate in this

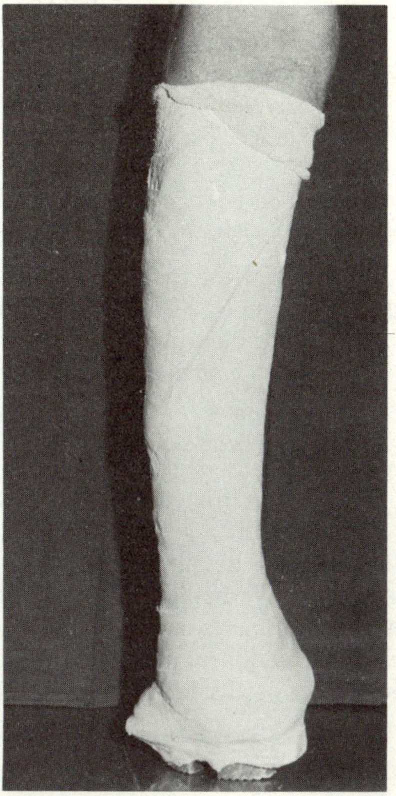

**Figure 9.6** Rigid plaster dressing with extension cork and rocker, Syme's level

type of IPOF due to the lack of space between the stump and the ground. In fact a Chinese rocker is much more effective in initial mobilisation.

At above-knee level suspension problems are considerable and the IPOF technique is not advocated.

The application of an IPOF requires considerable care and the correct materials are essential. It is not without risk to the inexperienced.

The advantages of rigid dressings are as follows.

1 Oedema is prevented from forming at the stump end, the wound healing more quickly.
2 There is less risk of infection since the dressings are applied in theatre and may be left undisturbed for 7–21 days.
3 The patient is more comfortable as the stump is not handled for bandaging, and as it is well protected the patient finds it easier to move in and out of bed. Pressure on the stump from bedding is avoided.

4 An extension tube incorporating a simple alignment unit can be attached to the plaster cast when mobilisation is intended. To this can be attached a prosthetic foot, enabling the more robust patients to begin early walking training.

### Nursing care of a patient with a rigid dressing—features of importance

1 Make sure the strap attaching the cast to the waist belt is taut when the patient stands but that it does not pull the stump into hip flexion.
2 Check the plaster dressing daily to make sure there is no excessive movement or pistoning which, if present, will allow distal oedema and possibly infection to develop.
3 Minimal blood staining through the plaster denotes that further wound drainage has occurred and is a good, rather than bad, sign.
4 Report any offensive odour from the plaster as it may indicate that infection is present in the wound.
5 Report complaints of pain to allow the doctor to decide whether analgesics are appropriate or whether further investigation, including removal of the plaster, will be necessary.
6 Record the patient's temperature, pulse, and respiration (TPR) accurately four-hourly, preferably orally, for as long as his stump is encased in plaster of Paris.

### **Controlled environment treatment** (Figures 9.7–9.10)

This form of treatment is essentially an air dressing, the stump being enclosed in a sterile plastic container (a Sterishield) with a control system which allows the air in the container to be pressurised, cycling between high and low pressures at specific predetermined timings. In addition the temperature of the air can be controlled. Following development at the British Research and Development Unit, Roehampton, the system is marketed by Cape Engineering (Inter Med).

This management of stump environment is applicable at all levels from through-knee distally to partial foot. The authors believe that it may eventually prove to be an 'ideal' environmental treatment but at present its value has not been fully assessed. It is of great interest inasmuch as it is related to the physical environment, making no attempt to treat the wound or the stump in any other way. It imposes a precise and controllable environment and this must be compared with that related to other forms of dressing. How much pressure is created by bandaging? What rise in temperature results from soft dressings? These factors are of considerable importance in amputation surgery associated with vascular disease.

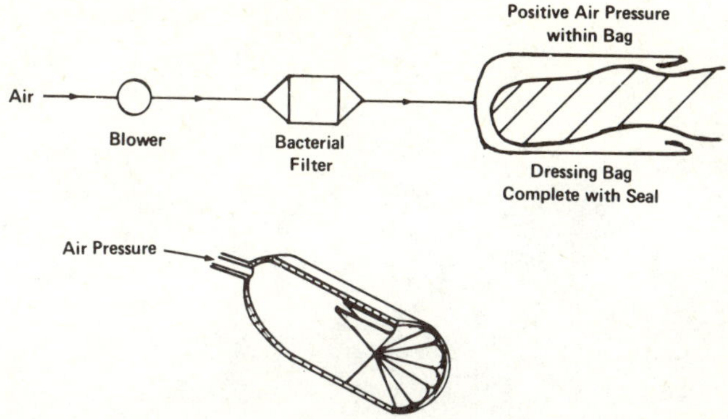


**Figure 9.7** Controlled environment treatment, basic principles

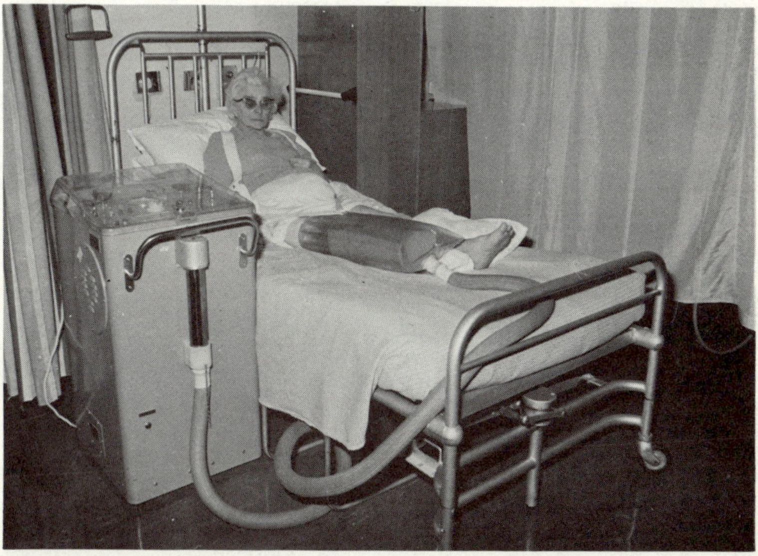

**Figure 9.8** Controlled environment treatment, below-knee patient undergoing treatment

There are very specific advantages.

1 There is no skill of application.
2 There is adequate control of pressures.
3 There is adequate control of temperature.
4 The dressing is sterile.
5 The stump can be observed.
6 The proximal joint, i.e. the knee, can be mobilised.
7 Oedema, post-surgical, is minimised.
8 There is no tourniquet effect or localised high loading on the tissues.

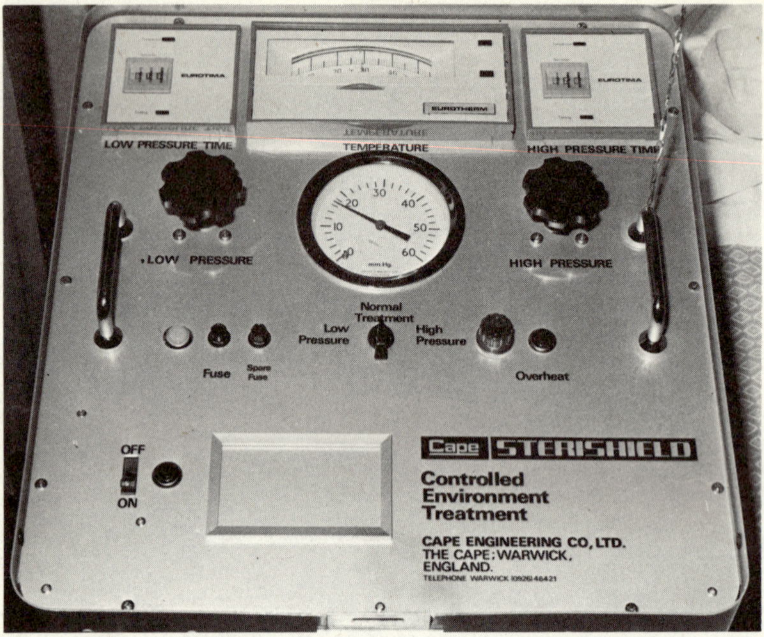


**Figure 9.9** Controlled environment treatment, control consul

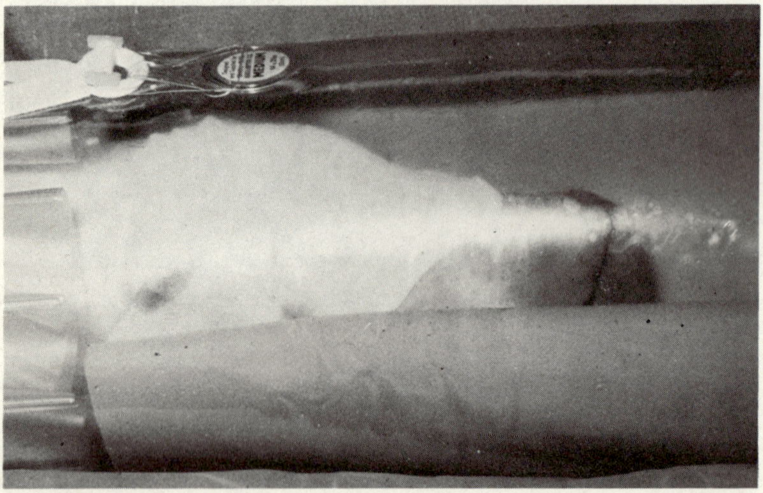

**Figure 9.10** Controlled environment treatment, below-knee stump in Sterishield

## The healed stump

When the wound is completely healed the patient should begin to care for the stump himself. He should wash it daily and dry it thoroughly. He should learn to handle it without undue thought. This process of familiarisation is important since the final functional result depends to a great extent on the stump itself.

The patient should be shown how to bandage his stump and should practise doing so; it must be bandaged firmly for the first three to six months, whenever the prosthesis is not being worn, e.g. at night. Oedema may arise at the end of the stump if this procedure is not followed, with resulting stump/socket interface problems.

**Stump bandaging**

Stump bandaging is the responsibility of the nurse. It is extremely important and considerable practice is needed in order to do it effectively. If the stump is incorrectly bandaged delayed healing may result with alteration in stump volume. When the prosthesis is supplied it may not fit due to this alteration.

Before starting to bandage, the nurse should confirm where the suture line is situated so that the technique she employs will encourage rather than hinder the healing of the wound. Normally the suture line is situated in a specific area of the stump as follows:

1 transverse posterior or vertical in an above-knee;
2 transverse posterior or vertical intercondylar in a through-knee;
3 transverse anterior in a below-knee;
4 transverse anterior in a Syme's.

In all but the through-knee there is a long and a short flap and the aim in bandaging is to stress the long to the short flap, thus easing any undue tension on the suture line.

A stump bandage is applied, working from the distal end proximally, as its object, apart from holding the dressings in place, is to prevent terminal oedema forming or to disperse it if it is already present.

Crêpe bandages are used:

1 15 cm × 9 m for hip disarticulation or a hindquarter amputation. (It will be necessary to sew together two 15 cm crêpe bandages to provide sufficient length);
2 15 cm × 4.5 m for above-knee or through-knee stumps;
3 10 cm × 2.25 m for below-knee stumps;
4 10 cm × 4.5 m for Syme's amputation.

*Bandaging for hip disarticulation and for hindquarter amputation*

If the patient is very thin the opposing iliac crest should be lightly padded otherwise the skin may be damaged by pressure. With the patient supine commence at the waist on the affected side taking the bandage across the abdomen and round the waist for one-and-a-half turns before applying a divergent spica over the wound, bandaging from behind forward. Each layer of bandage over the wound is followed by a turn circling the waist.

It is important that the spica covers the whole area firmly from the groin to the iliac crest otherwise any oedema present at the operation site will not be fully dispersed.

*Bandaging the above-knee stump* (Figure 9.11(a)–(e))

The suture line is usually on the posterior aspect therefore bandaging should commence on the anterior aspect of the stump.

Using a 15 cm crêpe bandage start on the anterior aspect of the stump, holding the end of the bandage with the thumb at the level of the inguinal ligament. Take the bandage firmly down the stump, over the centre of the extremity and up to the gluteal fold, fixing it there with the fingers; repeat this layer in reverse back to the inguinal ligament. Now bandage the stump from outside inwards, with oblique figure of eight turns covering the corners of the extremity, proceeding up the length of the stump to the groin. The tension of the bandage should be greatest distally, decreasing slightly as the bandaging continues towards the groin.

Turn the patient onto his side and with the hip in full extension pass the bandage over the iliac crest, across the abdomen, and round the waist, recrossing the bandage at the iliac crest and continuing over the groin. Repeat this last turn of bandage firmly, especially in the adductor area, in order to avoid a roll of fat forming which would hamper limb fitting. Any remaining bandage may be spiralled down the stump towards the stump extremity.

It is important that the tension of the bandage is greater at the distal end of the stump in order to disperse any oedema. If the bandage is too tight proximally serious damage may occur by increasing instead of decreasing the terminal oedema. Safety pins should be used to hold the turns of bandage in place at the waist and at the groin if required.

*Bandaging the through-knee stump*

The method is similar to that used for the above-knee stump. The whole length of the stump is bandaged, and at least one turn should be taken round the waist and over the groin.

*Bandaging the below-knee stump* (Figure 9.12 (a)–(d))

The suture line is usually on the anterior aspect therefore bandaging should commence on the posterior aspect of the stump. Using a 10 cm crêpe bandage start posteriorly at the level of the fibular head, holding the end of the bandage in place with the fingers. Take the bandage firmly lengthwise over the centre of the stump extremity and up to the tibial plateau, securing it there with the thumb. Now cover the medial and lateral aspects of the stump extremity firmly and secure these longitudinal layers by means of an oblique turn round the stump. (Note: circular turns are *never*

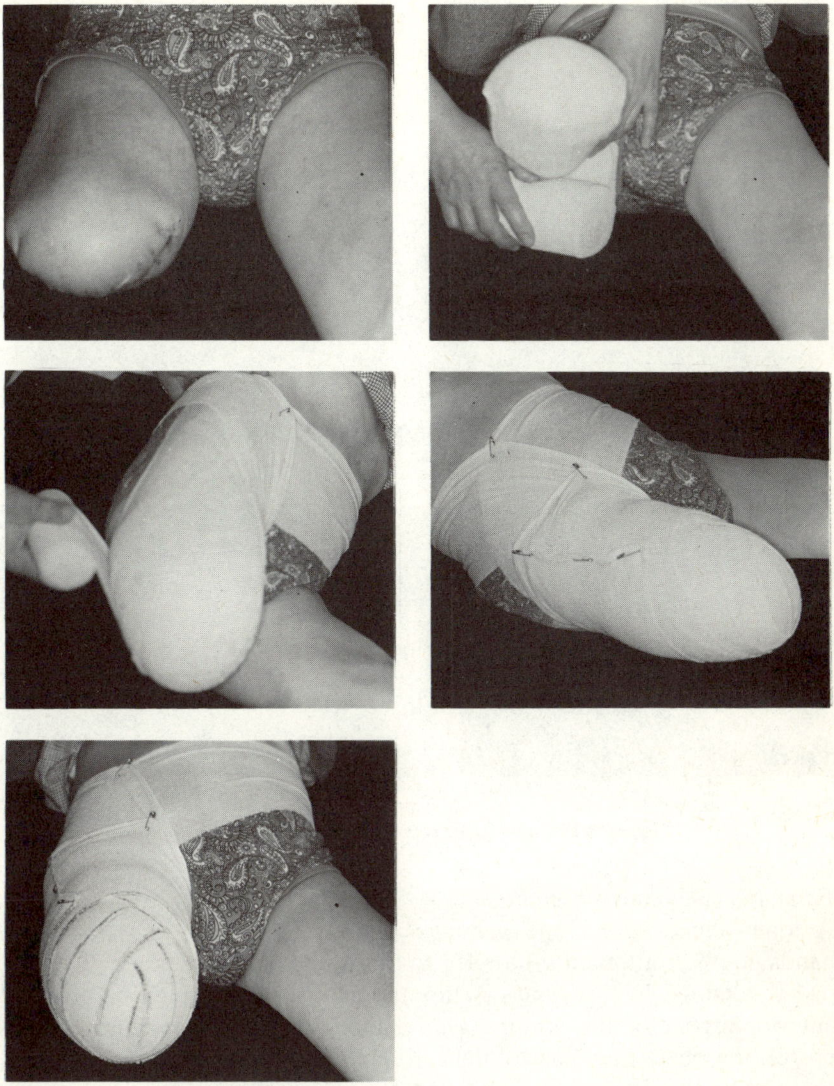

(a) (b) (c) (d) (e)

**Figure 9.11** (a)–(e) Above-knee stump bandaging

used on a stump.) Cover the sides of the extremity with figure of eight turns and proceed with these oblique turns up the length of the stump, gradually reducing the tension so that there is no undue constriction of the tissues. Avoid too many superimposed turns over the crest of the tibia otherwise the tissues may become devitalised. Complete the bandaging using two circular turns above the knee and pin securely. Remember the purpose is to achieve distal compression *without* any proximal constriction.

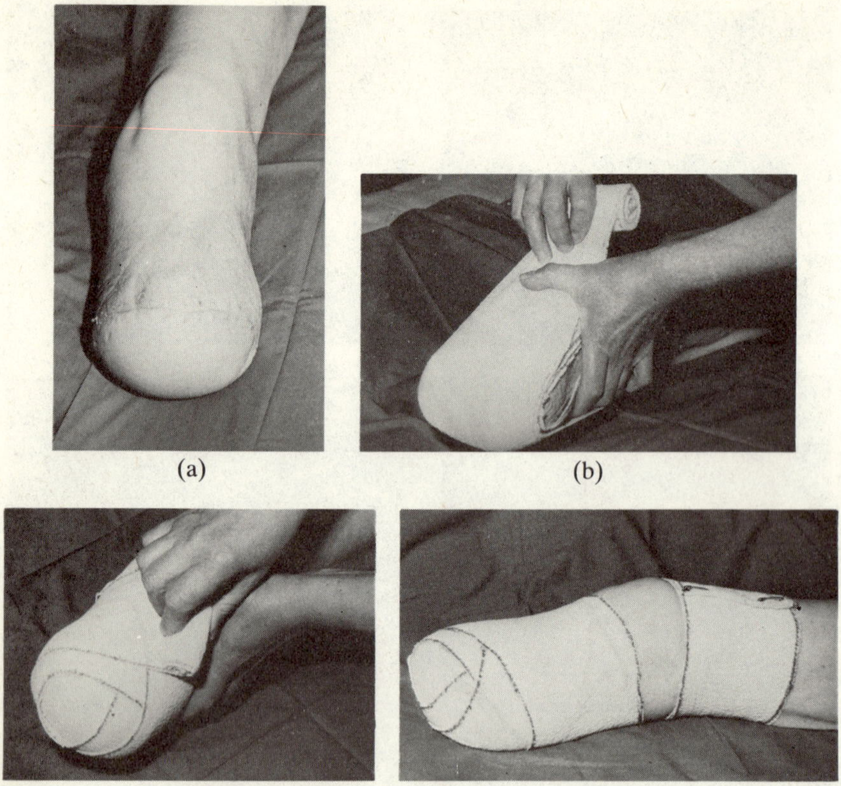

(a) (b) (c) (d)

**Figure 9.12** (a)–(d) Below-knee stump bandaging

*Bandaging a Syme's amputation*

A long 10 cm wide crêpe bandage is used because it is essential the bandaging be continued up the leg to finish just below the knee. The heel pad is retained in this type of amputation, the suture line being on the anterior aspect of the stump. Thus bandaging must commence on the posterior aspect of the base of the calf. Hold the end of the bandage firmly there with the fingers and proceed down longitudinally to the stump extremity and then up and over the suture line to half way up the tibial shaft, retaining the bandage there with the thumb. Now cover the lateral aspect of the stump, being careful not to cause any drag on the suture line when taking the bandage down over the corners of the extremity. Using oblique figure of eight turns, cover the stump from the extremity to just below the knee. Take care not to superimpose too many turns on the tibial spine and decrease the tension as the bandaging proceeds upwards. Fasten off the tail of the bandage below the knee.

Note: the basic aims of stump bandaging are:

1 distal compression;

2 the avoidance of proximal constriction;
3 the avoidance of high loaded areas, e.g. over bony prominences;
4 the avoidance of tight encircling turns of the bandage.

*Bandaging of partial foot amputation*

The general principle is to use a long 10 cm wide crêpe bandage, the method being very similar to that used for a Syme's amputation, the bandage being continued up the leg to finish just below the knee thus avoiding any 'waisting' effect. In the case of minimal forefoot amputations bandaging may be unnecessary or tubigrip support may suffice.

# 10 The Stump—Function and Associated Problems

## Function

The stump is the connecting link between the amputee and his artificial limb. It can be used functionally without the prosthesis to maintain balance, e.g. a below-knee stump can be hooked over seating or the bedside. When a Syme's amputation has been performed the patient is able to weight bear on the end of the stump and thus use it as a prop when dressing.

To enable the patient to walk comfortably again the stump needs to be strong, well healed, painless, and able to withstand the pressures exerted on it by the prosthesis. It is obviously less difficult for an amputee to walk if his operation has been performed below the knee for no mechanical knee can adequately replace the human knee.

Psychologically the more distal the amputation the less traumatic it is for the patient.

## Care of the stump

This is of vital importance since the patient's ability to walk in comfort will depend to a large extent on good postoperative care of the stump.

It is convenient to subdivide stump care into specific areas of interest as follows.

## Position of the stump

When the patient is in bed the stump should rest flat on the bed. A pillow must never be put under the stump as in an above-knee amputee it will cause hip flexion and in a below-knee amputee, knee flexion (Figure 10.1). Neither should a pillow be placed between the knees as this will cause abduction at the hip (Figure 10.2). The below-knee stump must not be allowed to dangle over the side of the bed and when the patient is sitting in a chair it must be supported on a stump rest, otherwise oedema will form and knee flexion may occur.

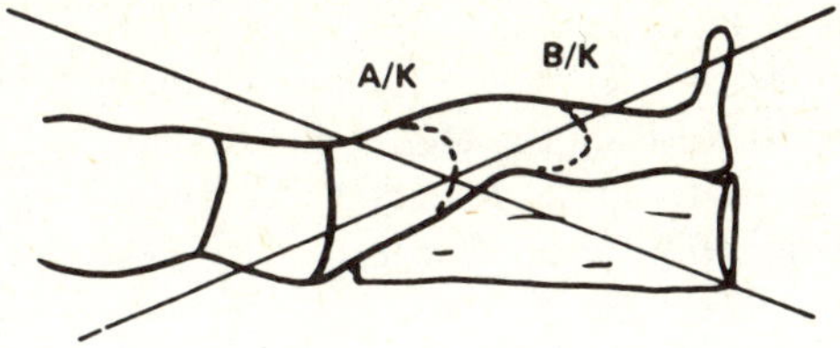


**Figure 10.1** A pillow must not be placed under the stump. A/K, above-knee; B/K, below-knee

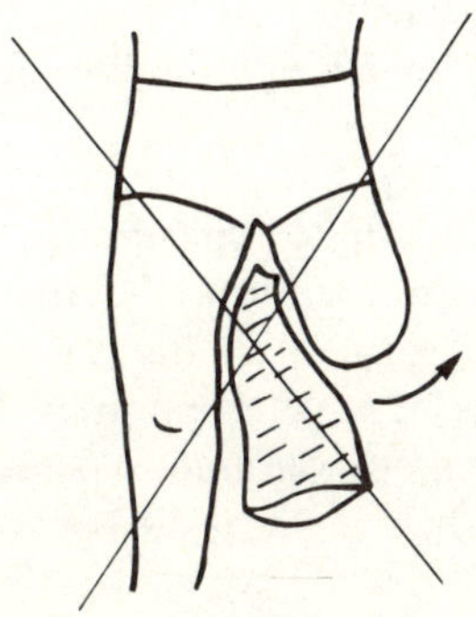

**Figure 10.2** A pillow should not be placed between the knees

## Wound drainage

Various methods are employed to avoid the formation of a haematoma at the site of operation. The more usual method is by continuous closed suction drainage into a bottle attached to the bedstead. It is extremely important that drainage does take place and, if it does not, the surgeon should be notified. Usually drainage has ceased after 72 hours, at which time the tube should be slowly and gently withdrawn. The drain fluid should be sent for bacteriological examination in order to determine the presence or absence of an infecting organism and the appropriate drug sensitivity.

## Stump pain

*Immediate postoperative pain*

Immediate postoperative pain will be relieved by an appropriate analgesic. If the pain persists it will be necessary to determine the cause. Generally, excessive pain is not a frequent feature.

*Persistent pain*

Persistent pain, difficult to relieve, occurring 24–72 hours after operation, may indicate the formation of a haematoma. This is a serious condition since, if it is not recognised and evacuated immediately, the increased tension will cause devitalisation of the tissues and a breakdown of the wound. When a haematoma has formed there is usually an increased pulse rate and a slight elevation of temperature.

*Pain due to infection*

Pain due to infection usually occurs during, or towards the end of the first week and is throbbing in character. It is associated with a raised temperature and an increase in the pulse and respiration rates. When infection is suspected it is necessary to inspect the wound, release any contained pus, and treat the infection with a suitable antibiotic.

*Pain due to a neuroma*

Pain due to a neuroma occurs much later but is less likely where the nerve has been severed under slight traction so that the cut end retracts into a bed muscle and the neuroma, formed by the natural healing process of the nerve, is protected. This type of pain may be felt during the third postoperative week. Repeated continuous percussion of the painful area may ease the condition but if the pain proves intractable surgery is required.

*Painful skin conditions*

Painful skin conditions may occur and will be secondary to the wearing of a prosthesis. The stump tissues are subjected to a completely new environment. They are compressed and are expected to bear high loads and often air is unable to circulate so that perspiration can result in problems.

Venous and lymphatic stasis may occur leading to terminal oedema. Capillary haemorrhage and crusting may occur with certain open ended sockets and suction limbs. This is known as distal congestion of the stump. Eczema may develop over the oedematous area.

Intertrigo may also arise in the groin and is associated with excessive perspiration and chronic irritation from the socket brim. A change in the type of socket or an adjustment to the socket and better support of the terminal tissues usually effect a cure.

Callosities may occur where pressure is taken on the ischial tuberosity and, in the below-knee amputee, on the patellar tendon and lateral aspect of the stump. This is in fact a protective response of the skin, enabling the amputee to weight bear more comfortably but occasionally proliferation of the tissues occurs resulting in a painful corn.

Contact dermatitis very infrequently arises after months of wearing a prosthesis and may be traced to one of the materials used in fabrication of the socket. The causal agent should be eliminated.

Epidermoid cysts can occur usually in an established above-knee amputee. The commonly affected areas are the inguinal and adductor regions and the ischial bearing area. These can become infected resulting in abscess formation which must be treated. Chronic cyst formation may require excision.

*Phantom pain*

Phantom pain occurs within the phantom limb, not in the stump itself. It is an abnormal sensation ranging from a slight tingling or numbness to the severe tearing or crushing pain suffered prior to amputation for trauma.

It is aggravated by scarring of the stump which might arise from infection, from a retained haematoma or where a painful neuroma has been caught up in the scar tissue.

Analgesics may give relief but in severe cases excision of scar tissue and neuroma with refashioning of the stump may be required. The patient's emotional state may influence the degree of pain, therefore tranquillising drugs may and frequently do provide relief.

**Phantom limb**

Perception of the phantom limb is strongest immediately following operation. It is considered normal for the majority of amputees to experience this phenomenon.

It is thought that an image of the absent limb is produced in the cerebral cortex through stimulation of the sensory nerve endings in the amputation stump. The body image must have been complete before there is a phantom limb therefore it could not occur where there is congenital absence of a limb. Strangely it does not manifest itself after Syme's or partial foot amputations.

The hallucination of the phantom limb can be so vivid that the patient may forget what is reality, namely the actual amputation, and attempt to walk without a prosthesis. Patients have been known to fall because of this, injuring the stump in the process, and therefore should be warned of this danger.

Firm bandaging of the amputation stump tends to lessen the sensation and gives some degree of comfort, as does wearing of a prosthesis.

Telescoping often occurs so that the phantom limb becomes progressively shorter, but the feet and toes, especially the great toe, continue to be felt for some considerable time. Usually the phantom limb, if painless, becomes an asset when the patient starts walking training as he feels he is using his own leg instead of an artificial one.

# 11 Prosthetic Replacement

The need for compensation for functional loss following amputation is obvious. There is a compelling demand to regain the facility to walk. Thus lower limb prosthetic replacement is an important subject, and all amputee care must be directed towards the final fitting and supply of a prosthesis. What are the essential characteristics of a prosthesis? Basically there are two elements which must be incorporated:

1 a well-fitting socket;
2 an alignment which would relate this socket correctly to the point of ground contact with the artificial foot.

Other essential factors are suitable artificial joints, some means of suspending the limb on a stump, devices to restrict excessive movement of the joints, and a total weight in keeping with the clinical requirements.

These considerations are aimed essentially at three aspects of special importance:

1 comfort,
2 cosmesis,
3 function.

These are of varying significance though all are necessary to every patient. In the young person function comes first, in the young woman perhaps it is cosmesis, in the breadwinner of the family, function, and in the elderly, comfort is the main essential.

Limbs are produced using a variety of materials, some due largely to custom and others following technological advances in the field of plastics in recent years. All materials have some special advantage: lightness, ease of use, satisfaction of design criteria, etc. Metal in the shape of dural, a lightweight alloy, is commonly used. Certain features, such as the incorporation of knee joints, require the use of steel, but this is kept to a minimum because of increased weight. The plastic in common use is a polyester resin laminate, incorporating stockinette and glass wool and forming a product of exceptional strength and durability. More recently carbon fibre has been considered as a means of adding strength but in the meantime its cost is excessive. Another material in use is wood; it may be used to produce a socket or it can act simply as a filler when using a plastic outer laminate. The wood commonly used for sockets is willow, being strong and easily worked. When acting as a filler, balsa is used for lightness. There are of course other materials, such as leather, other plastics, and rubber, used in various components of an artificial limb.

It is appropriate at this point to consider how a limb is constructed and fitted for an individual patient. As previously mentioned, the important task is producing an accurate socket. This may be done by simple measurement. However, if intimate fit is required a plaster casting

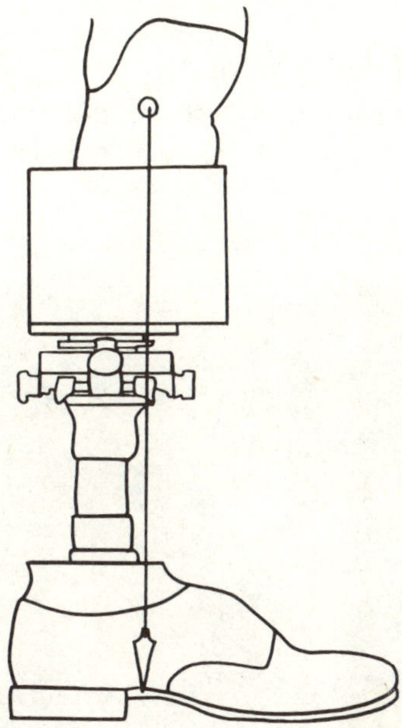

**Figure 11.1** Construction of a prosthesis showing an adjustable alignment jig

technique may be used. For example, consider a typical below-knee amputation stump. The prosthetist takes a plaster cast of the stump which reflects its shape and from this female cast a male model of the stump is produced, using liquid plaster mix. It is on this male model, following various rectifications, that the laminated plastic socket is fabricated. These rectifications are necessary because the prosthetist is aware that certain areas of the stump will accept pressure whereas others will not. By adding or removing plaster from the male model pressure can be avoided or created. The next part of the process involves the use of a vacuum bench, the plastic (polyester resin) in its fluid state being drawn into a stockinette and glass wool cover applied tightly around the rectified plaster model. The result is an extremely accurately fitting socket and on this the remainder of the limb is constructed. A fitting stage involving walking on an adjustable alignment jig allows the relationship of the foot to the socket to be established (Figure 11.1). This metal jig is later removed and replaced by balsa wood using a transfer jig to keep the socket and foot in the same position. Finally, after accurate shaping of the calf to match the remaining leg, an external laminate is applied to give the prosthesis strength and durability.

Specific levels of amputation demand varying types of prosthesis. There are many variations and clearly they cannot all be described in detail. However, it might be appropriate to describe replacement at varying levels.

**Through-hip prosthesis** (Figure 11.2)

The socket may be constructed in plastic or blocked leather and the basis of construction is a plaster model. It should be noted that there is a three joint replacement.

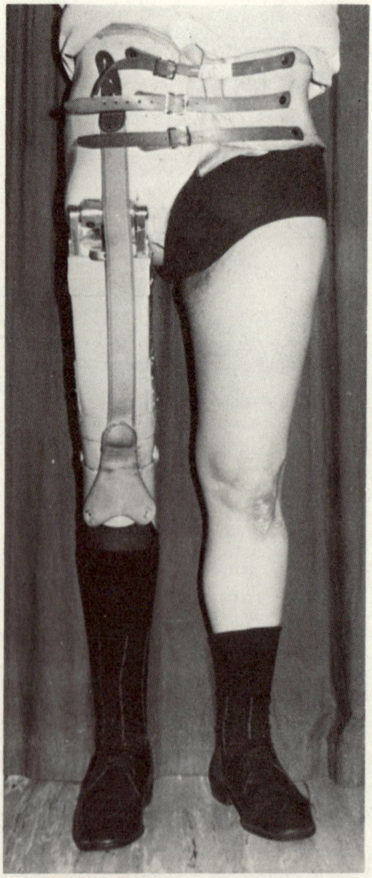

**Figure 11.2** Through-hip prosthesis

**Above-knee prosthesis** (Figure 11.3)

The sockets may have varying shapes, all based on some theoretical advantage, largely associated with expected comfort and function. Frequently they are produced in metal (dural) but plastics are also used in certain sockets. Suspension in the form of a pelvic band and shoulder strap may be necessary but need not be used in the suction socket, which is self-suspending.

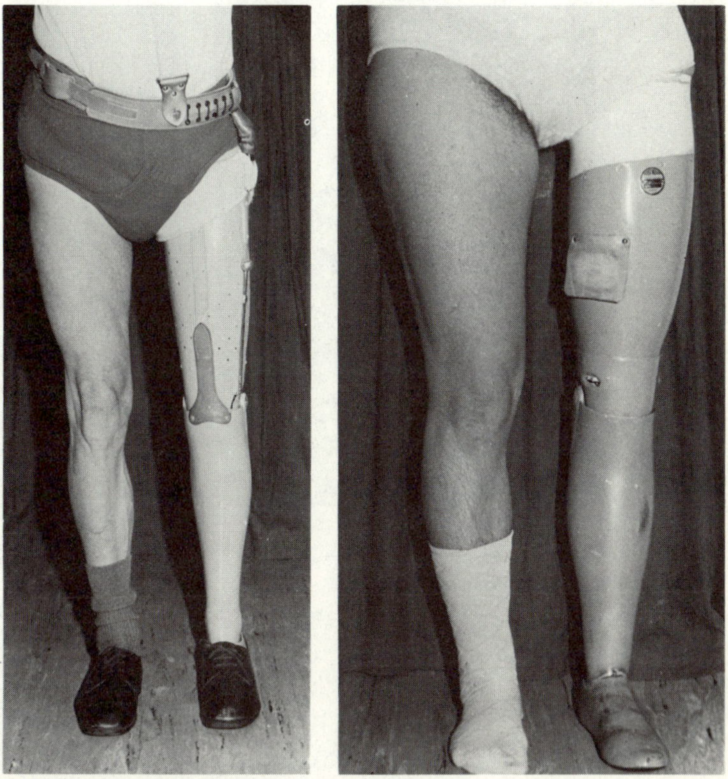

(a) (b)

**Figure 11.3** (a) Above-knee prosthesis, fabricated in metal. (b) Above-knee prosthesis, quadrilateral socket and suction suspension

**Through-knee prosthesis** (Figure 11.4)

The socket may be produced in metal, plastic, or blocked leather. The shape of the bulbous end created by the femoral condyles lends itself to self-suspension. Unfortunately an artificial knee joint, of necessity incorporated in side steels, in most cases leads to poor cosmesis around the knee. Experimental knee units are solving this problem and some, for instance four bar linkage systems, are available now (Figure 11.5).

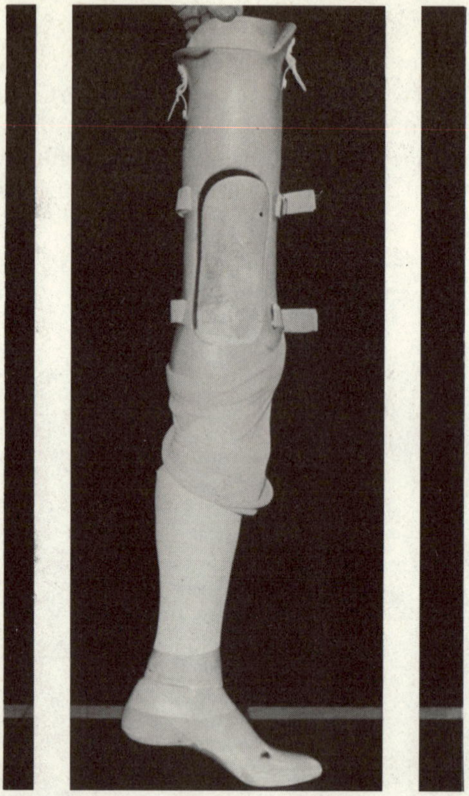

**Figure 11.4** Through-knee prosthesis, plastic socket with removable 'window' to allow entry of stump into socket

**Below-knee prosthesis** (Figure 11.6)

Almost all replacements at this level are made in plastic—the so-called PTB prosthesis (patellar-tendon-bearing). A large proportion of the weight is readily accepted on the patellar tendon and the fit is critical; changing stump volume (e.g. formation of oedema, weight increase or decrease) is obviously relevant. There are several variants of this type of prosthesis.

**Syme's prosthesis** (Figure 11.7)

The prosthetic design is created around the capability of this stump to accept end bearing. In addition the bulbous end is self-supporting. Plastic, metal, or blocked leather can be used in fabrication.

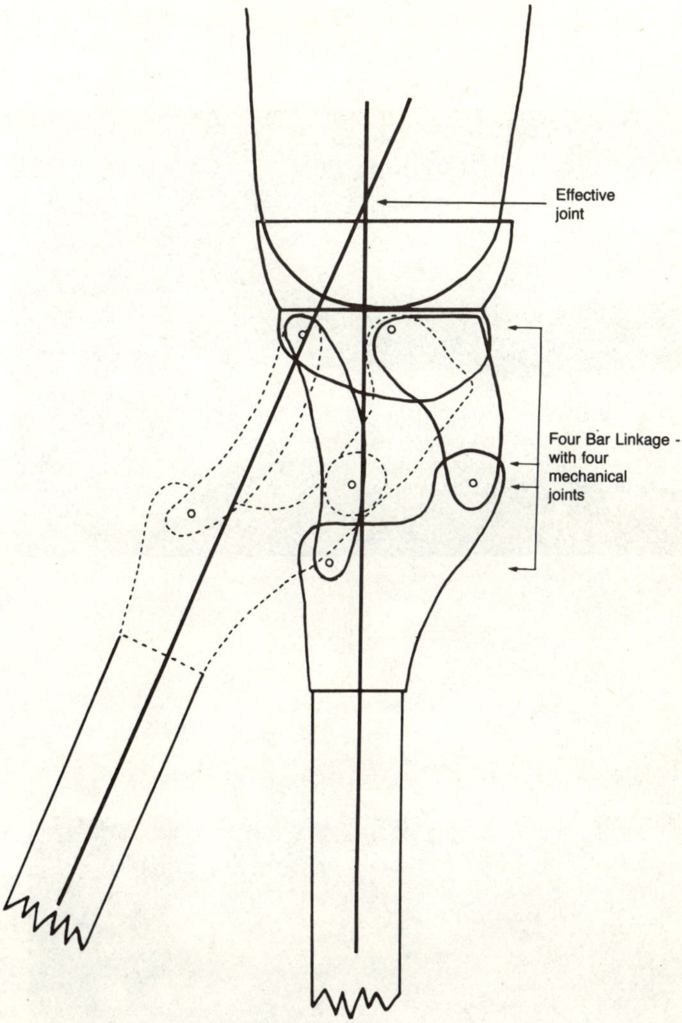


**Figure 11.5** Four bar linkage knee unit

**Partial foot prosthesis** (Figure 11.8)

By and large this degree of loss can be remedied by using a forefoot filler either in a normal shoe or in a special shoe or bootee.

**Modular assembly systems** (Figure 11.9)

Prosthetic fabrication for all levels of amputation has been undertaken for many years by various commercial firms. They have used well tried methods and conventional materials. The amputee has, over the years, gained much benefit.

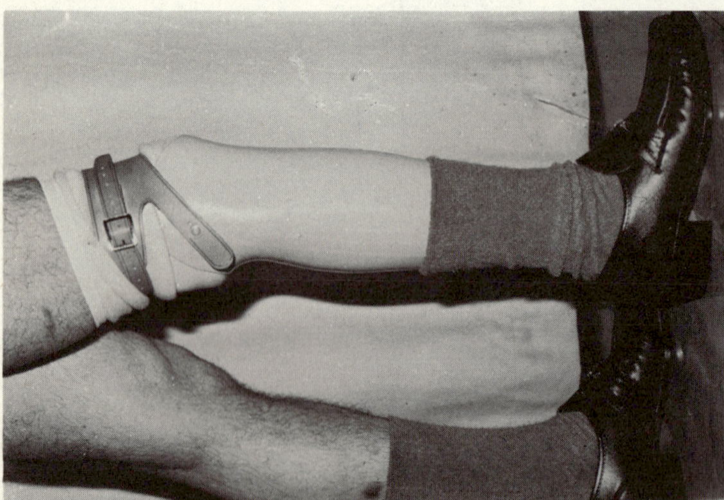

**Figure 11.6** Patellar-tendon-bearing below-knee prosthesis (PTB)

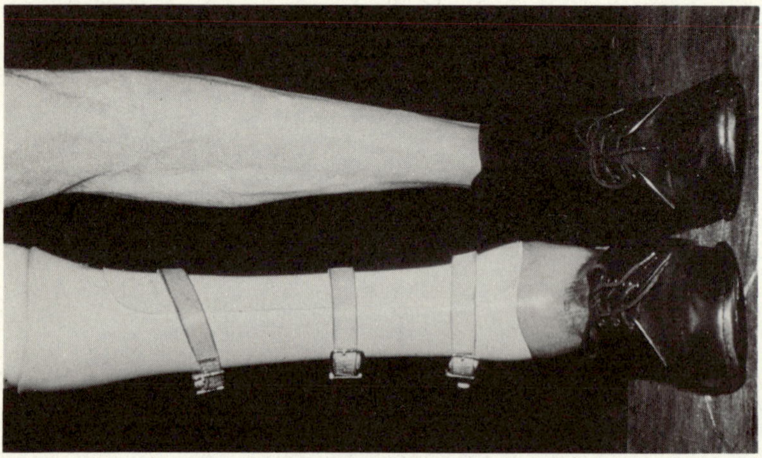

**Figure 11.7** Syme's prosthesis—plastic with 'window' to allow entry of bulbous stump

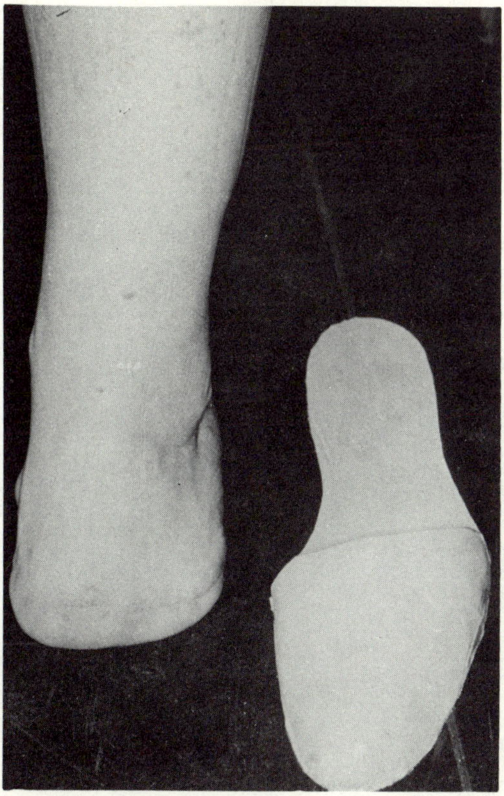

**Figure 11.8** Partial foot amputation with forefoot filler

In more recent years the limitations of this type of supply have been recognised. The inherent limitation of alignment potential, the relative delays seen in production and the lack of interchangeability of components have all assumed importance.

The modular assembly systems developed by various manufacturers throughout the world have rectified many of these limitations. Essentially they consist of off the shelf components which can be added to a custom made socket, allowing alignment and interchange of components as demanded by the clinical presentation. These components form the permanent skeletal structure of the prosthesis, simply requiring a soft covering or fairing suitably shaped to give a good cosmesis. The socket is generally constructed of contemporary materials such as laminates and thermoplastics. This system allows very rapid component replacement, e.g. new sockets can be added in two to three days, new knee units in less than one hour and replacement feet in even less time. The advantages are obvious.

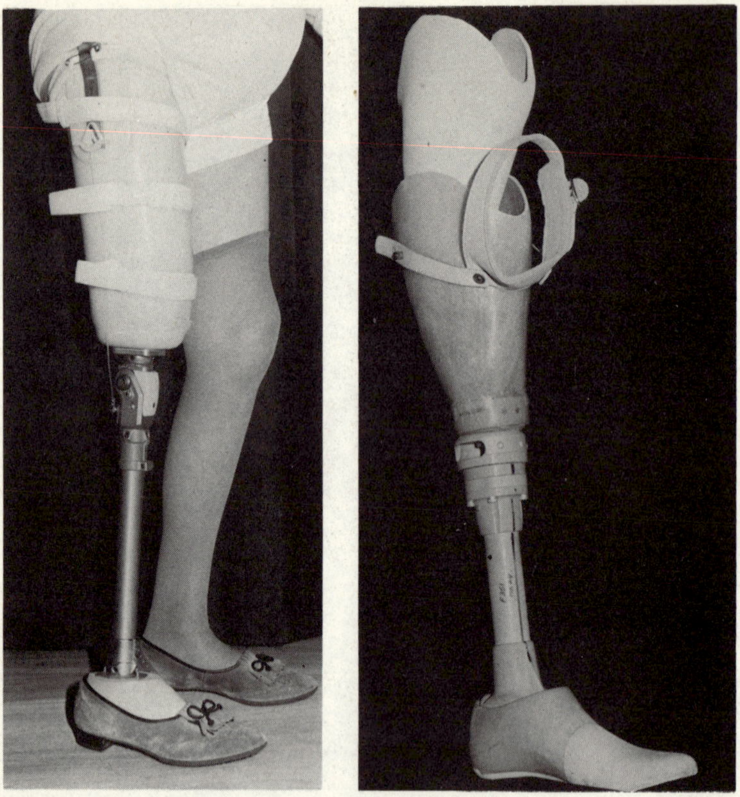

(a) (b)

**Figure 11.9** (a) Above-knee modular assembly system without cosmetic fairing. (b) Below-knee modular assembly system without cosmetic fairing

## Resulting function

The expected level of function depends upon many factors—stump, level of amputation, type of prosthesis, aids used, general medical condition, motivation, etc.

Generally, the higher the level, that is, the greater the loss, the less the expected function. However, some amputees at above-knee levels can still enjoy an active interest in sport, e.g. skiing, swimming, golf, etc. Below-knee levels allow a remarkable degree of activity and the best prosthetic users at this level are difficult to recognise as having lost a limb. One of the authors knows of a below-knee amputee, also suffering from total blindness, who very regularly indulges in weekend walks of 32–48 km in the Scottish mountains. Another amputee who has an above-knee loss spends his leisure time diving, using full aqualung equipment. Not all cases are in this category. It must be remembered that many of the primary amputees are in the older age groups; diminished activity is, of course, natural and quite acceptable in these cases, but even the older amputees can and do achieve a surprising degree of normality in walking ability for their age groups. Each case, old or young, must be judged on its own merits, and expected function, frequently in older people, becomes increasingly difficult to predict.

# 12 Technical Amputee Care

The amputee must be shown how to apply his prosthesis and how to care for it. He should be supplied with special woollen socks to fit the stump, except when a suction suspension limb, a hindquarter or a through-hip prosthesis is worn. In the suction limb the skin is in direct contact with the socket and in the hindquarter or through-hip clothing is used to protect the stump. If woollen socks are used a nylon or cotton sock may be worn beneath if there is any tendency for friction or excessive sweating. A clean stump stock should be used daily. When supplied, the woollen stump socks should be slightly larger than required as they tend to shrink a little with repeated washing. Shrinkage is minimised by washing them in hand-warm water containing well dissolved soap flakes, and then rinsing them thoroughly to remove and traces of soap. They should be carefully dried, avoiding direct heat. Nylon and cotton socks do not shrink and can be washed in hot soapy water, rinsed, and hung up to dry.

## Applying the artificial limb

The technique of applying the prosthesis will depend on the level of amputation and the type of prosthesis issued. Patients with peripheral vascular disease may have had bilateral amputations and this complicates the problem.

Consider each level in turn.

### **The hip disarticulation and hindquarter prosthesis** (Figure 12.1)

The prostheses for these extensive operations are somewhat similar in that each consists of a 'bucket' seat and a limb which is jointed at the hip, and ankle. The 'bucket' seat in blocked leather or plastic may be padded for comfort. Since no sock can be worn the amputee pulls his underclothing down smoothly over the stump as protection. The limb is applied whilst standing and held in place by straps at waist and hip levels.

### The above-knee prosthesis

The above-knee pylon (Figure 12.2) is a temporary prosthesis, fabrication

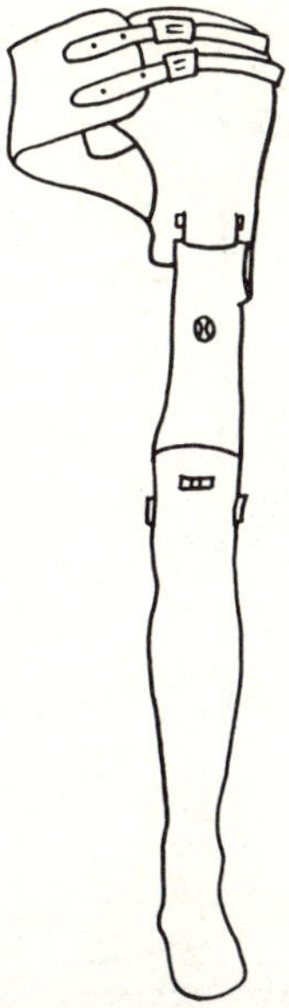

**Figure 12.1** Hip disarticulation and hindquarter prosthesis

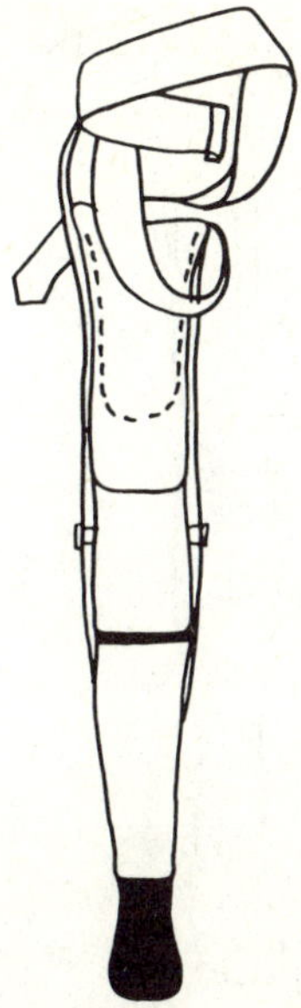

**Figure 12.2** The above-knee pylon

being possible in two to three days. It is lighter than an artificial leg, reasonably easy to apply but, although functionally permitting early mobilisation, it is not aesthetically pleasing.

It consists of a rocker end, metal side steels hinged at the knee, and a metal socket shaped to allow ischial seating. It is held in place by a pelvic band with a shoulder strap suspension.

The elderly amputee usually lies on his bed to put on a pylon. The woollen stump sock is pulled over the stump, the stump being placed in the socket with the pylon externally rotated. The sock is pulled up higher and its edge is turned down over the socket brim. The pelvic band is tightened which has the effect of aligning the pylon correctly by rectifying the external rotation. The shoulder strap is brought over the opposing shoulder and attached to the front of the pelvic band. The more modern type of above-knee prosthesis may incorporate an adjustable quadrilateral plastic socket with modular components including a Sach foot. The application is essentially the same, the socket adjustment having been previously determined by the prosthetist.

The conventional above-knee prosthesis (Figure 12.3) is applied over a woollen stump sock. The method of applying it is similar to that used for the pylon.

The suction type of prosthesis (Figure 12.4) may have a plastic, quadrilateral, total contact socket or a metal socket, and occasionally it may be total surface bearing in design. It requires neither a pelvic band nor

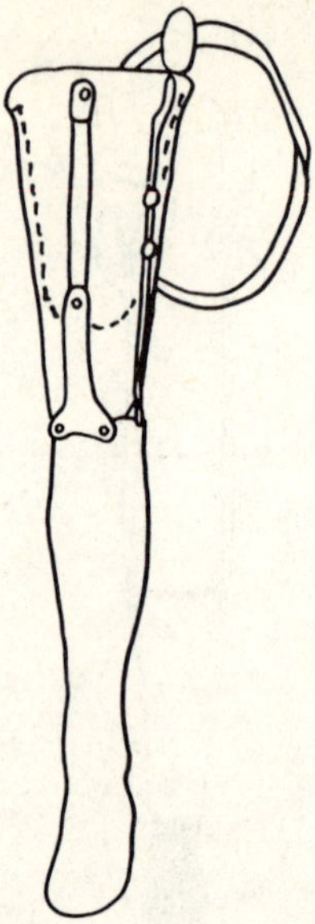

**Figure 12.3** The conventional above-knee prosthesis

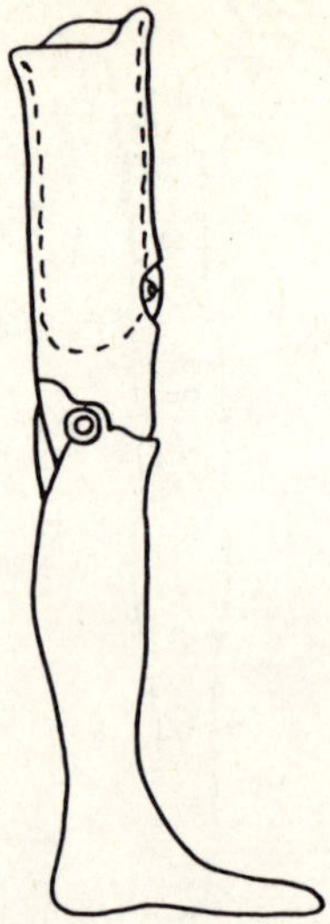

**Figure 12.4** The suction type of prosthesis

a shoulder strap, being suspended by the suction created by the intimate stump/socket fit; no stump sock is used. The prosthesis must be applied while standing.

A length of 15 cm crêpe bandage is spiralled down the stump from the groin to the extremity, and the end of the bandage is pushed out through the valve hole in the socket. The stump is inserted into the brim of the socket and, whilst weight bearing, the amputee eases or 'milks' the stump into the socket by pulling the bandage down through the valve hole until complete withdrawal of the bandage is achieved. The stump should then be *totally* enclosed by the socket. The valve is fixed in position and functions by allowing air to leave the socket but not to enter.

**Bilateral above-knee amputees**

Patients may be supplied on a temporary basis with short 'rockers' (Figure 12.5). These consist of rocker ends, side steels and sockets with a short pelvic band combined with shoulder straps to give suspension. Their height varies from 45 to 60 cm. They are usually put on as a pair, i.e. laced together at the back where the hemipelvic bands meet.

In order to apply short rockers the amputee sits on his bed with the 'rockers' in front of him, the rocker ends resting against the end of the bed and externally rotated. Having pulled on his stump socks he eases himself forward over the pelvic band until he can place his stumps in the sockets.

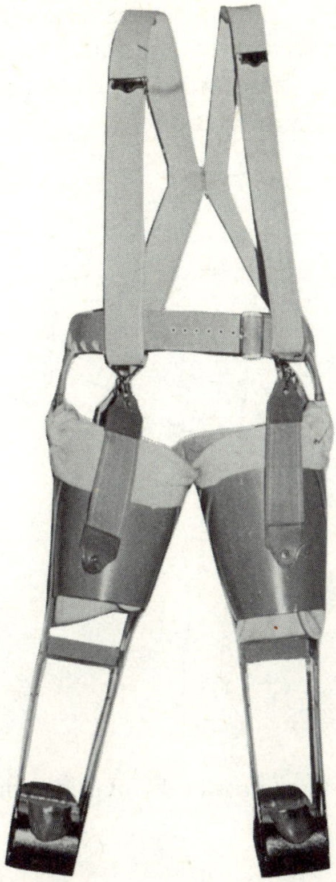

**Figure 12.5** Short 'rockers'

He then lies down and pulls the back of the pelvic band up over the buttocks, at the same time easing his stumps further down into the sockets. He slips his arms through the shoulder straps and fastens the pelvic band and in doing so aligns the prostheses. The tops of the stump socks are then pulled down over the rim of the sockets.

**The through-knee prosthesis** (Figure 12.6)

Although the shank of this limb is produced in metal with side steels incorporating knee joints, the socket may be of several types—blocked leather, plastic with a removable window, or metal. These all use the end bearing potential of the stump.

The stump is protected with a woollen sock (through-knee size), placed within the thigh corset, or through the plastic socket brim, whichever applies, and then the amputee stands so that the stump extremity rests firmly on the end bearing pad incorporated within the socket. He now pulls up the sock towards the groin and either laces the corset, clips the plastic window in place, or fastens any suspension fitted to the limb. The leather and plastic sockets are self-suspending and the metal socket, which requires suspension, is a straight plunge fit.

Finally, the upper edge of the stump sock is eased down over the rim of the prosthesis to prevent skin friction.

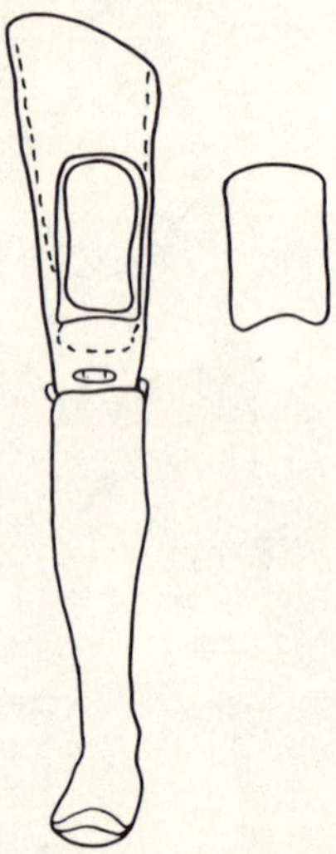

**Figure 12.6** Through-knee prosthesis, plastic with removable 'window'

## The below-knee prosthesis

Various types of prostheses are available for this level of amputation.

*The patellar-tendon-bearing (PTB) prosthesis* (Figure 12.7)
This is probably the quickest and easiest to apply. The amputee sits on a chair or bed and pulls the suspension cuff or knee strap forward over the front of the socket. The stump, with its stump sock smoothly in place, is slipped into the socket and then the amputee either stands in order to locate the stump accurately within the socket, or exerts pressure whilst seated. The knee strap is then pulled up over the patella and fastened securely round the supracondylar region of the lower thigh. The Fajal variant of the PTB prosthesis does not require a knee strap since the prosthesis is suspended by the socket extending above the patella (Figure 12.8).

The Fillauer type of socket also avoids the use of cuff suspension (Figure 12.9). It relies on a special shaping of the medial wall of the socket, which extends above the medial femoral condyle holding the socket securely in position. This can be achieved either by using a suspension wedge which fits above the condyle inside the socket, or by a removable part of the socket with special supracondylar shaping in this area.

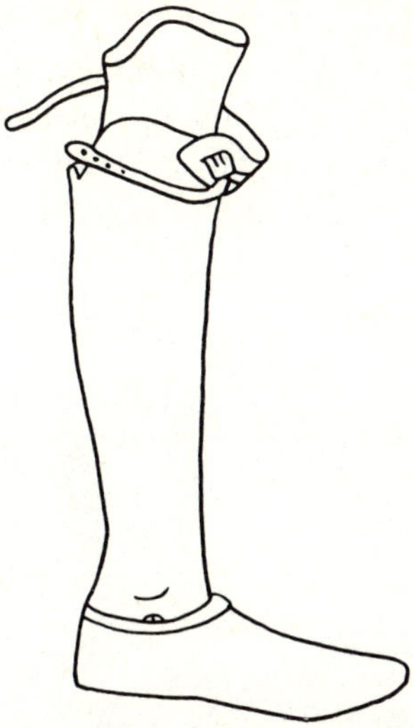

**Figure 12.7** The PTB prosthesis

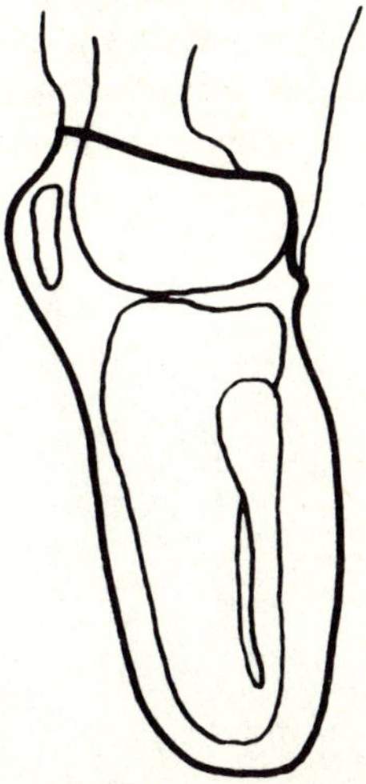

**Figure 12.8** Fajal or PTS socket, enclosing and being suspended by the patella. PTS, prothese tibial supracondylienne

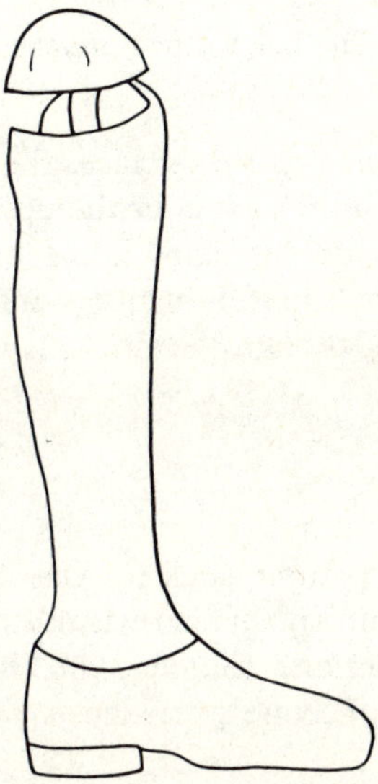

**Figure 12.9** Fillauer or KBM socket, supracondylar suspension. KBM, Kondylen Betting Munster

*The below-knee prosthesis with thigh corset* (Figure 12.10)
The leather thonging of the corset is loosened and the stump with its long woollen sock is passed down to position itself within the socket. The amputee now stands, pulls up the stump sock as far as it will go and

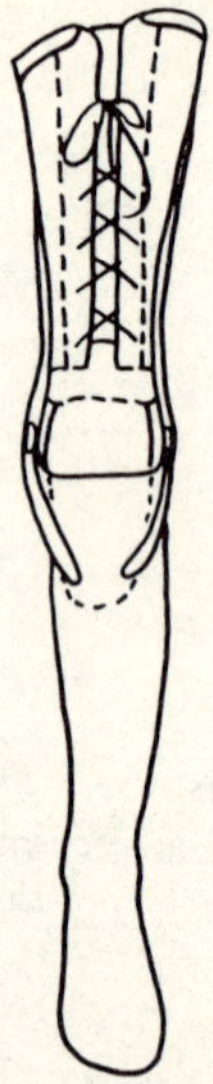

**Figure 12.10** The below-knee prosthesis with thigh corset

keeping his weight on the prosthesis, laces the thigh corset firmly. He then eases the edge of the stump sock over the upper rim of the thigh corset so that no friction occurs on his skin. Some elderly amputees find it less difficult to lace the corset loosely whilst standing and then to tighten the laces after sitting down, though the fitting is less precise when the limb is applied in this manner.

**The Syme's prosthesis**

An appropriate woollen stump sock for this level of amputation is pulled on firmly over the stump so that no wrinkles remain to irritate the skin. The sock has a bulbous end shaping, the fit being intimate. There are several different types of Syme's prosthesis.

*Open Syme's* (Figure 12.11)
The stump is pushed inside the prosthesis until it rests on the end bearing pad and the blocked leather gaiter is laced up firmly.

*Metal enclosed Syme's* (Figure 12.12)
The stump is placed in a removable blocked leather socket and then both

socket and stump are thrust inside a metal (dural) container; the leather socket is then attached to the container by elasticated clips.

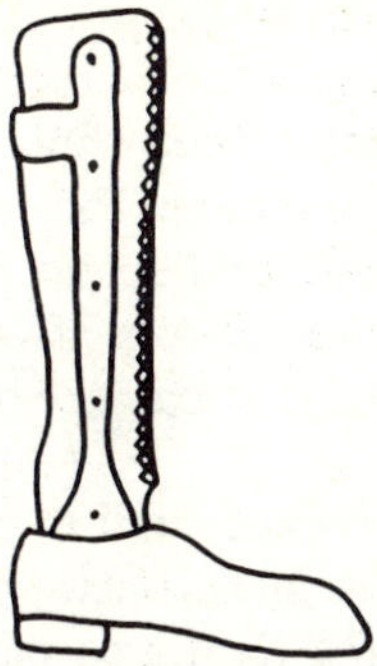

**Figure 12.11** Open Syme's prosthesis

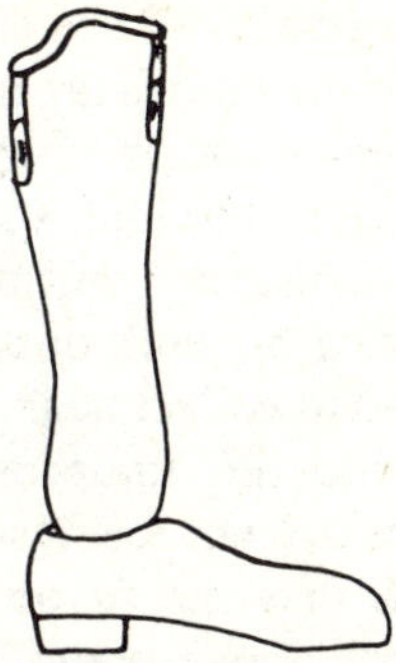

**Figure 12.12** Metal enclosed Syme's prosthesis

*Plastic Syme's* (Figure 12.13)
This type has a removable window in the side of the laminate, the aperture of which is wider than the stump extremity. In order to apply the prosthesis the stump is placed through the proximal end and then extended out

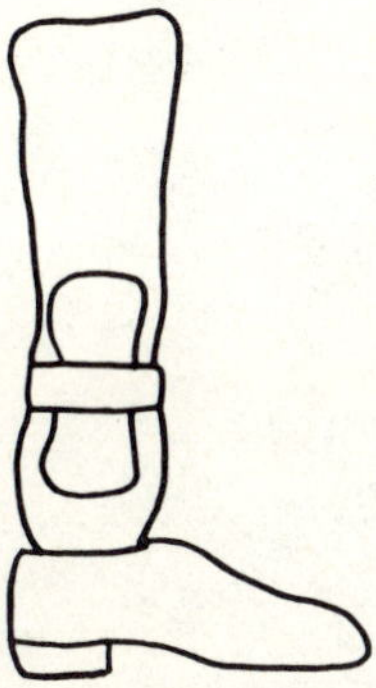

**Figure 12.13** Plastic Syme's prosthesis

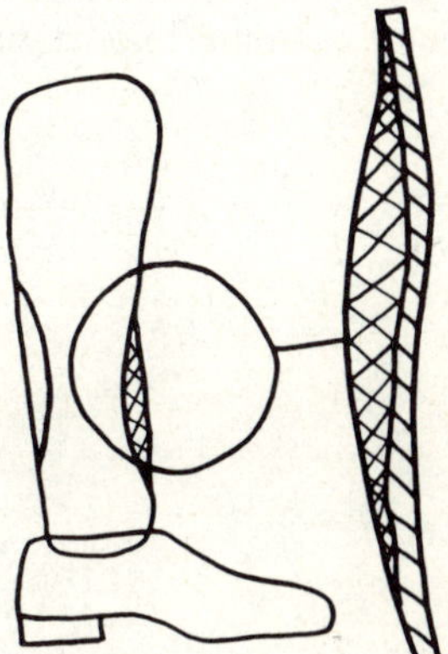

**Figure 12.14** Plunge fit Syme's prosthesis

through the window and placed down and back through the window into the bulbous base of the prosthesis. The window is then fitted back in position and the encircling straps are fastened.

*Plunge fit Syme's* (Figure 12.14)
This prosthesis has an inner liner of rubber and fine leather which is applied to the stump, both then being 'plunged' into the plastic laminated container.

## Care and cleanliness of the prosthesis

Amputees must be taught how to look after their artificial limb or limbs and a daily routine should be established from the beginning. At the end of each day when the limb is taken off, the socket should be wiped out using a clean cloth rinsed out in soapy water, and then dried thoroughly. The external surface of the limb should receive similar care. The joints should be kept dry to prevent rusting and this should be kept in mind if the amputee is using his limb outside in wet weather. Pieces of wool or fluff may, if allowed to collect near joints or knee locks, impair the operation of these parts, rendering the prosthesis unsafe.

Padding should not be inserted into the socket of the limb—if the amputee feels that the fit of the prosthesis is unsatisfactory he should request an early appointment at his Limb Fitting Centre so that examination and any necessary adjustments can be carried out.

Since the amputee has a duplicate prosthesis it should be used in rotation; if not, it may seem uncomfortable when required. This duplicate prosthesis is supplied so that the amputee always has at least one serviceable limb available and there should be no problem in sending a damaged or worn limb in for repair.

Artificial limbs, although expensive, are essential for the amputee if he is to continue his independence and therefore their correct use and maintenance is of extreme importance.

# 13 **Abnormalities of Amputee Gait**

Normality, as far as one can judge it, has been described, and clearly any departure from this pattern amounts to abnormality. We can all recognise some very basic abnormalities of gait, but it is not quite so simple to determine the cause purely on casual observation. The cause can be very minor (a tiny stone in one's shoe leading to acute discomfort), or major (a leg discrepancy reaching anything up to 20 cm). It may be caused by other components of gait—an abnormal range of motion of a joint or a weakness or incoordination of a muscle.

In the amputee we have a slightly different situation inasmuch as we have three components or factors which may be at fault: first, the stump and second, the prosthesis itself. The third factor is the patient, his build, physique and any environmental factors involved (Table 13.1). At this stage remember the relative inadequacy of man to replace a human limb with a device constructed in metal, wood, leather, or plastic. Even in this highly technological age, nothing approaching true replacement can be achieved. At the same time it must be said that with some artificial limbs, the skills of the prosthetist and the patient are such that in many cases normal gait can be achieved.

**Table 13.1 Main causes of abnormal amputee gait**

| *Stump* | *Prosthesis* | *Patient* |
|---|---|---|
| Pain | Ill-fitting socket | Habit |
| Flexion deformity | Bad alignment | Attitude |
| Muscle weakness | Incorrect length | Motivation |

## The stump

Abnormalities of the stump must be considered as possible causes of gait deviations. It is not commonly the site of pain but it is possible that pain, either from pressure or movement associated with the socket of the prosthesis can be a limiting factor. More frequently the problem exists in or around the joint immediately proximal to the amputation level, as it may be the site of a fixed flexion deformity. This type of deformity can often be accommodated within the prosthesis but it may present an insoluble problem (e.g. at the knee). The range of function may be limited by muscle contracture resulting in adduction, abduction, or flexion deformities. Equally these deformities may be due to other causes—joint capsule involvement or skeletal abnormality. It is of importance, even within the context of this chapter, to emphasise the part good nursing and skilled therapy, pre- and postoperatively, can play in the prevention of these deformities.

The efficiency of any stump depends largely on its strength and this, in turn, depends on the residual muscle left after operation and the actual operative technique. It is easily appreciated that muscles correctly trimmed and attached under tension to the bone end of a stump will result in better function. The prosthesis is in itself non-functional—the stump and its muscles are the power-house controlling its function.

There are other factors associated with the stump. An adductor roll of flesh above the socket brim, often leading to painful cysts; the formation of a neuroma, which of course is always present when a nerve is sectioned and may, if superficial, be painful; an excessively prominent bony structure and factors associated with the skin and its reaction to wearing a limb—all these can cause abnormal gait deviations.

## The prosthesis—What part does it play?

There are, in fact, only two elements of crucial importance in a prosthesis—the socket and its alignment. The socket is self-explanatory; the alignment is simply the relationship of the socket 'in space' to the ground. If both of these factors are correct, the limb should function—it may not be cosmetically acceptable, and this is another important consideration. The socket must fit, some more intimately than others, and it must be comfortable. Sockets are designed and produced on well tested criteria. It is not simply a question of sticking a cork (i.e. the stump) in a bottle. There are certain parts of the stump which would object very strongly to being asked to accept the load of weight bearing, and there are others which accept pressure without complaint. The alignment, as has been said, means the set-up or construction of the limb perhaps through one or two joints between the socket and the ground (Figure 13.1). This is quite critical and prosthetists may spend many hours aligning a limb to suit the patient's particular manner of gait. This does not mean to say that they introduce such elements as valgus or varus deformity at the knee—this would be impossible in a mechanical device even if it was an attempt to match cosmetically the patient's remaining leg. The precise way in which this alignment is carried out need not be described, but suffice to say it is

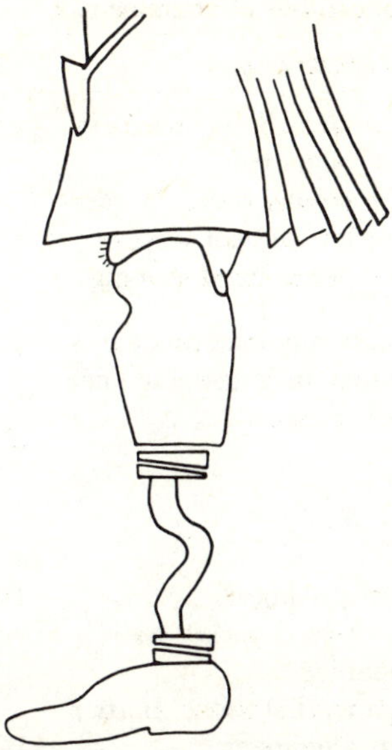

**Figure 13.1** Alignment showing importance of relationship between the socket and the ground regardless of intervening hardwear

highly technical and quite essential in the production of a limb. Given a good socket and accurate alignment gait deviations are minimised.

One further element in prosthetic design should be mentioned—the weight of the limb. This varies from material to material and clearly must vary according to the patient's needs. The vigorous young man needs a more sophisticated limb which is able to withstand heavy use. The older person would find this type of limb a burden and quite unnecessary. It should be said that nearly all prosthetic replacements are in fact lighter than the natural limb, although it is difficult to convince some amputees that this is so: authorities are currently directing their attentions to this problem. Heavy and light duty limbs should become accepted practice in the future and this should be of great benefit, particularly for the geriatric amputee.

## The patient

The patient presents problems not associated with either the stump or the artificial limb. Abnormal build and physique, as in a non-amputee, produces gait deviations. State of mind also plays a part in the production of a gait pattern. It is well known that the studied, careful gait in the clinic is normally a change of pattern for the individual concerned. Factors, both intrinsic and extrinsic, play a part in building a pattern, whether it be

**Table 13.2 Recognised abnormalities of amputee gait**

| *Deviation* | *Prosthetic causes* | *Amputee causes* |
|---|---|---|
| Abducted gait | Excessively long prosthesis<br>Poor alignment<br>High medial socket border<br>Poor lateral wall shaping<br>Poor pelvic band shaping | Abducted stump not recognised by alignment<br>Habit |
| Circumducted gait | Excessively long prosthesis<br>Inadequate prosthetic knee involvement | Abducted stump not recognised by alignment<br>Weakness of stump and fear related to knee flexion |
| Lateral bending trunk | Short prosthesis<br>Poor lateral socket wall shaping<br>High medial socket border<br>Poor alignment | Defective balance<br>Abducted stump not recognised by alignment<br>Painful stump<br>Short stump<br>Habit |
| Rotation of prosthetic foot on heel strike | Excessive resistance to plantar flexion of foot<br>Poorly aligned foot<br>Poor socket fit | Forced extension of stump at heel strike to induce safety<br>Defective muscle control of stump |
| Terminal swing impact (rapid forward shin movement leading to forced full extension) | Insufficient knee braking<br>Excessive extension assistance | Positive attempt to achieve full extension prior to heel strike |
| Foot slap | Insufficient resistance to plantar flexion | Thrusting prosthesis onto ground to ensure extension |
| Uneven heel rise | Insufficient resistance to knee flexion<br>Insufficient extension assist at knee | Flexor/extensor muscle imbalance in stump |
| Vaulting—rising on toe of 'good' foot to ease swing on prosthetic side | Long prosthesis<br>Poor suspension—less of stump/socket relationship<br>Limited knee flexion | Fear of stubbing toe<br>Walking faster than prosthesis will allow<br>Habit |

Abnormalities of Amputee Gait

| *Deviation* | *Prosthetic causes* | *Amputee causes* |
|---|---|---|
| Uneven arm swing | Poor socket fit giving pain | Poor balance<br>Fear or habit |
| Uneven timing (short prosthetic stance phase) | Imbalance of knee action<br>Unstable alignment<br>Poor socket fit giving pain | Weak stump<br>Poor balance<br>Fear |
| Long prosthetic step | Fixed flexion stump not reflected in alignment of socket | Fixed flexion deformity beyond prosthetic alignment adjustment |
| Unstable prosthetic knee | Knee centre aligned forward of weight line<br>Poor socket alignment<br>Excessive resistance to plantar flexion of foot leading to delay in forefoot contact with ground | Hip flexion contracture<br>Poor hip extension power |
| Medial and lateral heel whips—at beginning of swing phase | Excessive knee rotation<br>Excessively tight socket —stump rotation reflected at heel | Habit |

normal or abnormal. The individual's way of life, his attitude to the disability, his profession, the area in which he lives, all play some part. Distinct abnormalities of gait may develop because of these factors, but, perhaps of more importance, the initial walking training tends to set its mark on the future. It may be good, bad, hurried, or perhaps even absent.

The recognised abnormalities of amputee gait are described briefly in Table 13.2, without going into detail of all the causes.

Abnormal amputee gait is clearly a complex problem but it is an extremely important aspect of total amputee care. If, as seems likely, specialist teams are created in the future, it is mandatory that all team members should be familiar with such abnormalities and that they should have adequate training and prosthetic orientation.

# 14 **Physiotherapy**

Regardless of the expertise of the surgeon, physician, or prosthetist, it is relatively useless to fit an artificial limb and offer no advice or training in its use. This is the province of the physiotherapist and on her treatment depends the final result of amputation surgery and prosthetic fitting. Ideally the physiotherapist dealing with amputee care should have particular training in this special field.

Early mobilisation and ambulation avoids complications such as deep venous thrombosis. Naturally this is of even greater importance in the primary amputee by virtue of the nature of the condition necessitating treatment. For this reason patients should seldom remain in bed for more than a few days following amputation, being initially mobilised in self-propelled wheelchairs. This immediately widens interest and, as well as being psychotherapeutic, it involves the use of the upper limbs which are important for additional support in the early stages of formal walking training.

At first, routine postoperative physiotherapy should be carried out and during the early rehabilitation period the physiotherapist should direct her efforts to bed exercises (Figures 14.1–14.3). The patient should be taught active stump exercises as soon as possible to maintain and improve joint mobility and muscle strength. These should be built up gradually to resisted exercises, particularly for the extensor groups. The importance of this cannot be overemphasised.

The danger of flexion deformities has been stressed and it is at this early stage that they may develop. It may be necessary to encourage the patient to lie prone for a short period twice a day with his pelvis flat on the bed, thus resisting the tendency to flex. This may be contraindicated in certain medical conditions and depends on the patient's fitness.

Physiotherapeutic measures must also be directed at concurrent functional defects, e.g. a pre-existing hemiplegia or stiffness of a joint due to arthritic change. This treatment is intended to prepare the patient for formal walking training when the prosthesis is fitted and to create an optimum level of acceptance of that training.

There should follow, early in the second postoperative week, continuing treatment in the physiotherapy department consisting of work between walking rails (Figure 14.4). It is important that walkways are designed

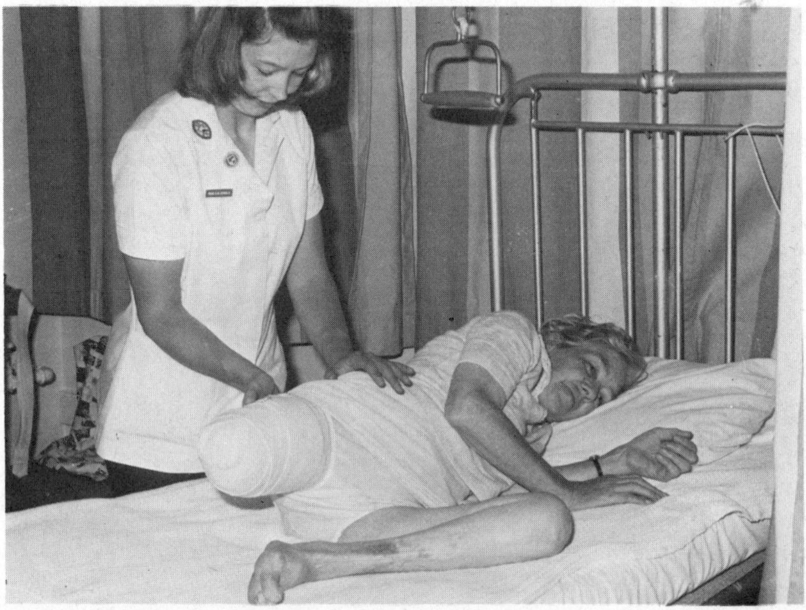

**Figure 14.1** Bed exercises

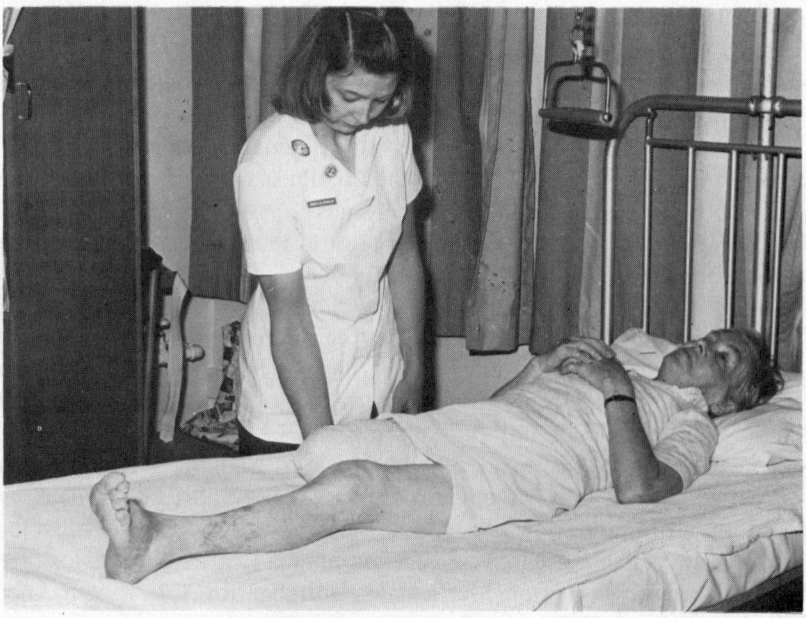

**Figure 14.2** Bed exercises

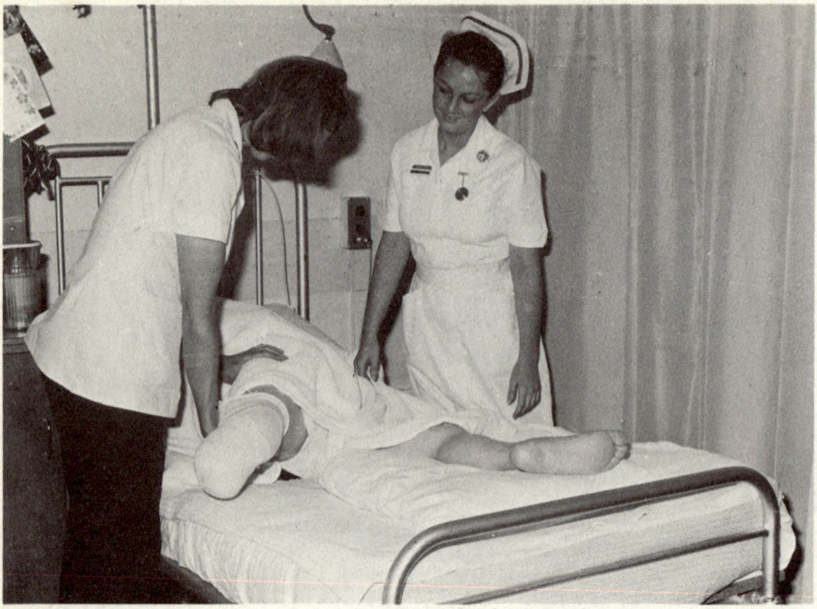

**Figure 14.3** Bed exercises

correctly, giving hand rails of correct dimensions and height in an area which is long enough to allow the patient to develop a normal manner of progression. The length should be at least 10 m and full length mirrors should be positioned at each end. The physiotherapist can then indicate gait and postural defects to the patient, who may recognise and correct any abnormalities. In addition at a later stage female patients are able to appraise the cosmetic appearance of the prosthesis, and this may be almost more important than function in some cases.

Reorientation may be necessary and prior to the fitting of the prosthesis, standing between rails using the remaining leg as the only support point is essential.

There follows hopping between rails using the remaining leg for support. This activity is beneficial and also accustoms the patient to the resumption of the erect position. By the time the prosthetic fitting is carried out the patient, therefore, is already partially mobile.

More recently it has been possible to start walking training at the preprosthetic stage using a pneumatic type of support. Known as the pneumatic postamputation mobility aid (PPAM aid), following development by the British Research and Development Unit, Roehampton, it is marketed by Vessa (Inter Med). It is suitable for long above-knee, through-knee, and below-knee stumps. In use, plastic envelopes are inflated to act as a socket for the stump and pressures of 20–40 mmHg are imposed increasing to 60+ mmHg when weight bearing. The plastic

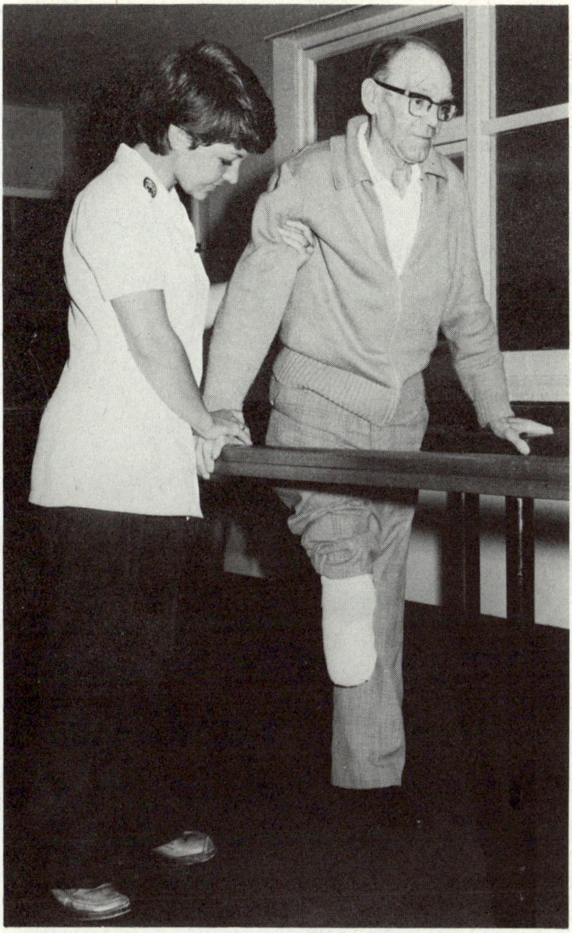

**Figure 14.4** Practice with walking rails

envelopes are attached to a metal frame (with proximal suspension for the very short above-knee stump) and a distal extension to a rocker end (Figure 14.5). In the younger person mobilisation on crutches would naturally replace the use of walking rails.

Following prosthetic fitting the first stage of activity is again within rails—at first standing and obtaining balance, then moving the body slightly from side to side and to and fro thus 'getting the feel' of the new prosthesis. Although spatial orientation is achieved by the eyes with the hands providing support on the walking rails, there is a feedback from the stump and the joint proximal to the amputation level. As prosthetic use increases so does the stump feedback become more effective.

The natural progression from walking rails is to sticks, at first in walking rails and later outwith this walking area, depending upon the patient's

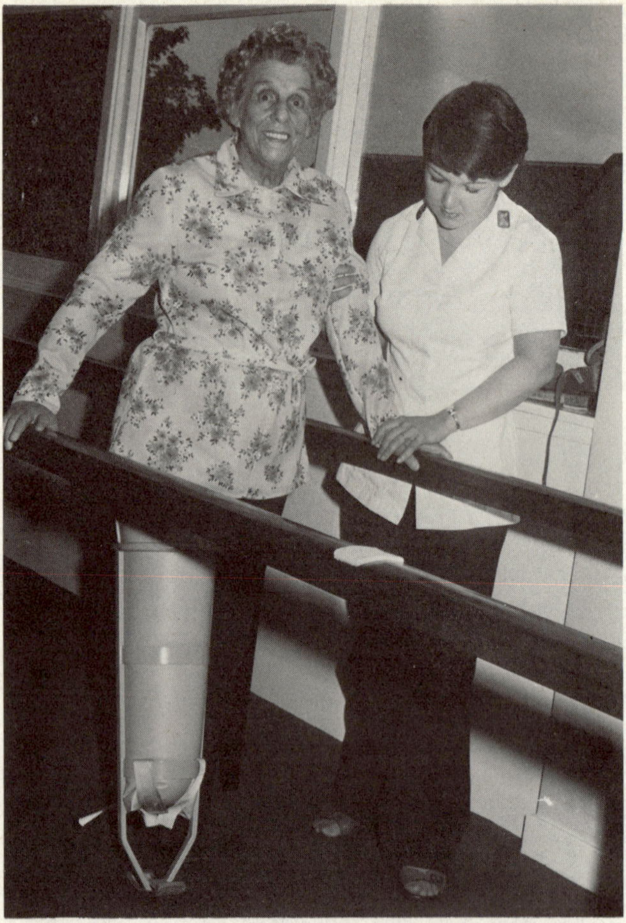

**Figure 14.5** PPAM aid

ability. Finally, it is to be hoped that only one stick held in the contralateral hand will be necessary (Figure 14.6). There are of course variations, largely dependent on age, concurrent disabilities, and perhaps social requirements. It may be that the very old patient with an amputation may require the stability afforded by a walking frame (Figure 14.7). This mobility aid used in domestic surroundings can be awkward; it is bulky and furnishings may leave little space. However, its use is considered perfectly justifiable if only to afford security. It may be that a walking frame will allow the patient to stand at the cooker or sink with greater confidence, thereby increasing the sense of independence. The use of a walking stick may depend upon the ability of the patient to grip the handle firmly. In this context Fischer sticks are useful, incorporating a moulded plastic hand grip which reflects the contours of the palm and thenar eminence. This

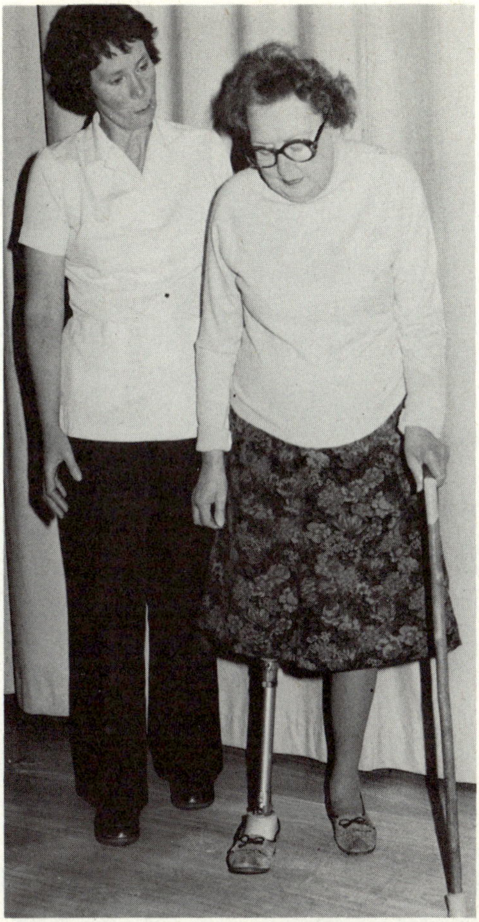

**Figure 14.6** Walking with a stick in the contralateral hand

increases the patient's ability to use a stick rather than a quadrupod, the latter only being considered in the frail patient.

Apart from individual training the amputees should have group physiotherapy in order to improve their general and physical conditions, thereby increasing their mental alertness and ability to integrate socially.

It is important to teach an amputee how to rise from and sit down on different types of chair, how to get up from the floor should he accidentally fall, and how to ascend and descend stairs.

**To sit down on a chair** (Figure 14.8)

The amputee faces the chair and pivots his sound foot until the back of his leg touches the chair. He then bends forward at the waist, allowing the sound hip and knee to flex thus lowering the trunk into the chair.

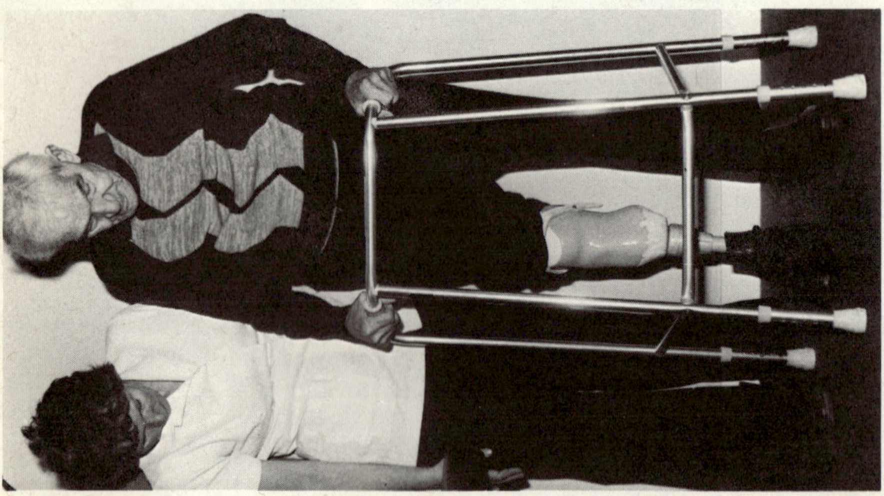

**Figure 14.7** Walking with the aid of a walking frame

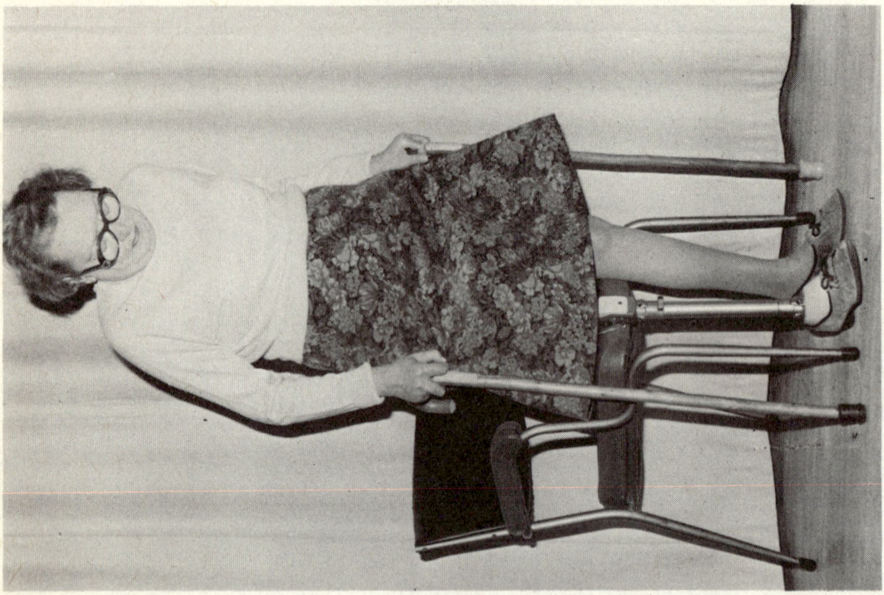

**Figure 14.8** Learning to sit down on a chair

**To rise from a chair** (Figure 14.9 (a) and (b))

The amputee places the sound foot close to the chair, grasps the arm rest, bends forward at the waist and puts the weight onto the sound foot and rises by extending the sound hip and knee.

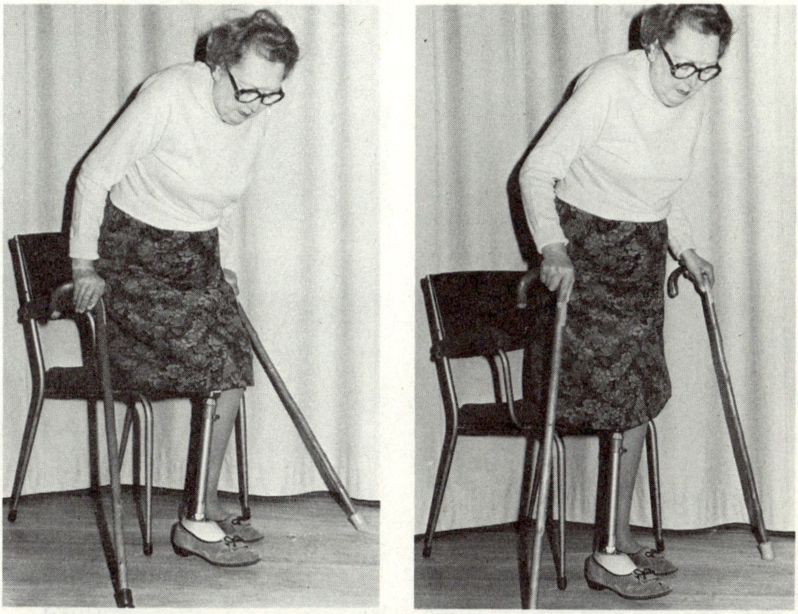

(a) (b)

**Figure 14.9** (a) and (b) Rising from a chair

**Rising from the floor** (Figure 14.10 (a)–(d))

The elderly amputee usually needs assistance to do this, or he may crawl to a strong piece of furniture and use this as a support. Alternatively, he should bend the sound knee and bring the foot under the trunk; place the hand on the sound side behind the trunk; turn towards the sound side, pushing with the hand while extending the sound leg and pivoting on the sound foot so that the opposite hand is also on the floor; push with both hands to extend the sound knee; bring the prosthetic foot level with the sound foot and extend both knees.

**Ascending stairs** (Figure 14.11)

This usually presents no problem to the below-knee amputee who is able to take alternate steps first with the sound foot and then with the prosthetic foot, although initially the method is similar to that used by the above-knee amputee. The above-knee amputee puts the sound foot on the first step and transfers his weight to that leg, he extends the hip and knee and in

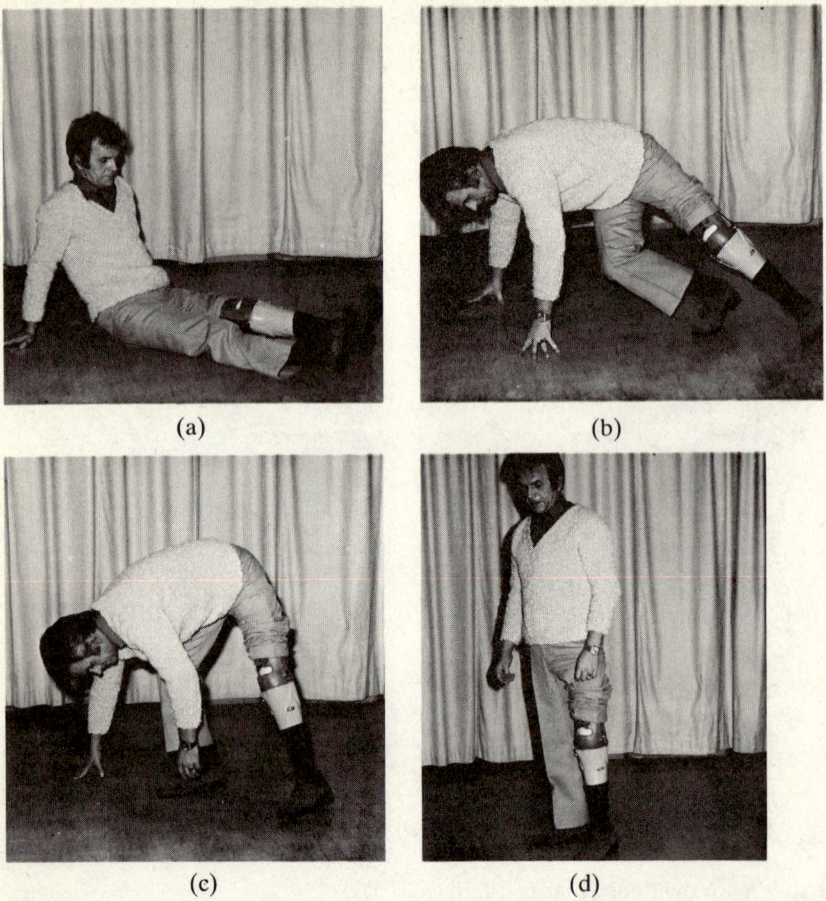


**Figure 14.10** (a)–(d) Rising from the floor

doing so brings the prosthetic foot up on to the first step alongside the sound foot. The sound foot leads to the next higher step and again the prosthetic foot is brought up to it.

**Descending stairs** (Figure 14.12)

The prosthesis leads to the next lower step and the sound leg follows to join it on that step. The weight is then transferred to the sound leg and the prosthesis is lowered by flexing the sound hip and knee, the weight then being transferred to the prosthesis, and the sound leg is lowered.

The bilateral amputee has, of course, far greater problems to face than the single amputee. So much depends on physical fitness and on the level of amputation. A bilateral above-knee amputee is unlikely to have the sheer physical strength and stamina to use full length prostheses but, if reasonably fit, may be trained to walk on short rocker pylons (Figure

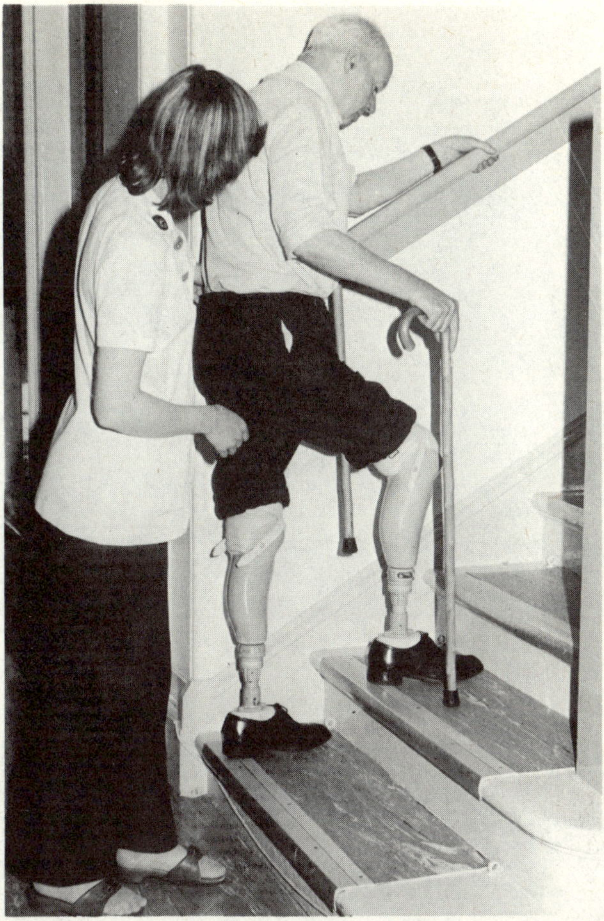

**Figure 14.11** Ascending the stairs

14.13). A warning should be given that height will be very much reduced when wearing these prostheses, but they will enable some degree of independence in the home to be achieved and balance will be more positive. The bilateral below-knee amputee will in all likelihood be able to live independently again.

The ideal environment for a Centre caring for amputees will include the facility to experience walking on varying surfaces, e.g. cobbles, rough gravel, tarmacadam and grass (Figure 14.14). In addition short inclines and declines, not only in the line of progression but directly across it as seen in many city pavements, should be negotiated. Steps and stairways, indoors and out, should also be included. Short visits outwith the Centre, e.g. to shopping areas, are beneficial.

The walking training already described may have taken place using a

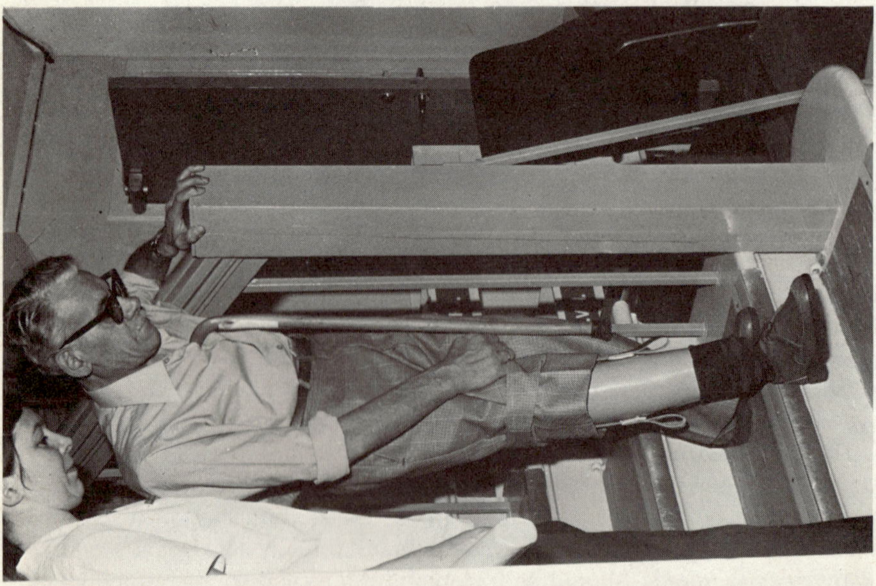

**Figure 14.12** Descending the stairs

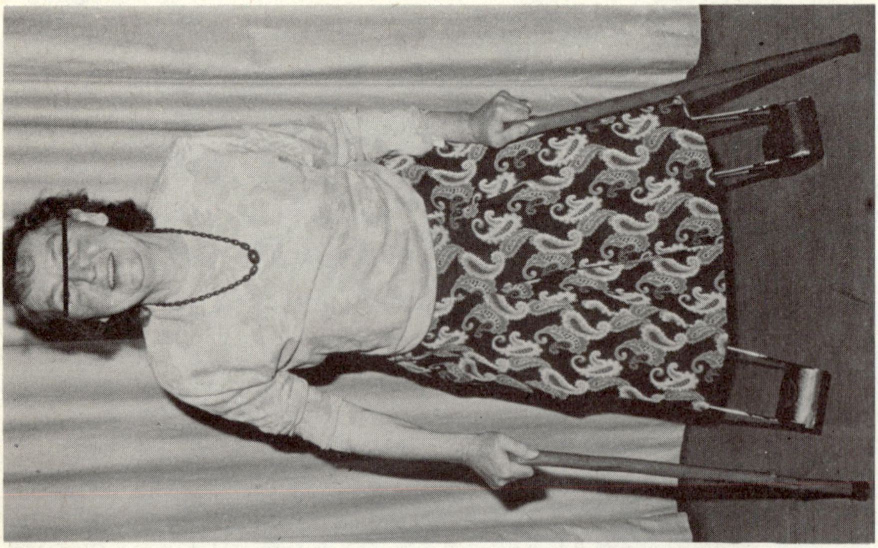

**Figure 14.13** Learning to walk on short rocker pylons

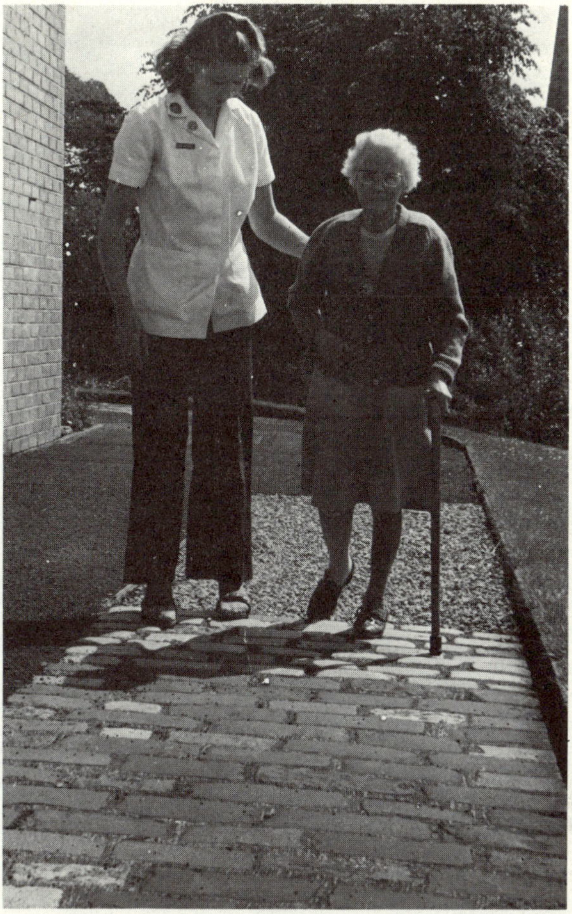

**Figure 14.14** Gaining experience of walking on varying surfaces

temporary prosthesis not incorporating a knee, ankle unit or a prosthetic foot, e.g. a temporary pylon. It is therefore necessary to follow up the delivery of the second or definitive limb with further training. The patient must be taught how to use the limb, adjust the knee control, correctly applying the various supporting or restraining straps, and clear the prosthetic foot when walking. All these activities are best carried out as an inpatient, perhaps utilising a hostel type bed rather than a bed with full nursing care. It should be remembered that Limb Fitting Centres are mainly regional and the distance from the patient's home may be such that outpatient training is impracticable. Finally, during continuing care, the physiotherapist must be involved in correcting defects of gait which have developed for one reason or another. It may be a bad habit brought about by an ill-fitting socket, or a stump problem. The physiotherapist acquires a special knowledge of these matters and, along with the prosthetist who should be immediately available, she can arrange for any rectification of the limb considered necessary.

The primary amputee population in the United Kingdom tends to consist of older people; this is inevitable by virtue of the nature of the causative disease. It is our view that age itself is no bar to training and it should be remembered that even minimal activity in a person in the middle eighties can perhaps enable a return to a domestic situation which is far preferable to long term care in a hospital or welfare home.

## Summary of gait training using prosthesis

### Below-knee level

*In parallel bars*
Standing
Posture/stance adjustment
Balance exercises
Rhythmic stabilisation
Exercises: marking time
flexion } knee
extension } knee
prosthetic foot forward, bear weight until foot flat with knee flexed, reverse until knee extended
as above, over, good foot to prosthetic foot

### Above-knee level

*In parallel bars*
Instruction on operation of knee lock (if present)
Standing, feet apart, check level and prosthetic suspension
Exercises: balance
gradual reduction of hand support
pelvis, pushing laterally and anteriorly, prosthetic side, resisted
weight shifting, pelvic movement only
(a) feet together
(b) prosthetic foot forward
(c) good foot forward
hip hitching, prosthetic side
good side

**All cases**

*In parallel bars*

Three point gait: hands/prosthesis/good leg (pelvis forward, stump back, never stoop to avoid adductor corner pain in above-knee case)

Four point gait: right hand/left leg/left hand/right leg (may be difficult with the elderly)

Maintain posture/weight bearing/equal steps

Use one stick

Use two sticks

*Out of parallel bars*

Use two sticks (a)

Use one stick (b)

No aids (c)

Possible acceptance of (a), (b), or (c)

Possible acceptance of Zimmer

*Specific training*

Negotiating rough surfaces

Ascending/descending stairs

Ascending/descending inclines

Clearing obstacles

Self-protection when falling

Rising from floor

Picking up objects

Kneeling/rising

# 15 **Rehabilitation in Activities of Daily Living (ADL)**

It is obvious with the lower limb amputee primary training is mainly concerned with ambulation under varying conditions and concerns the physiotherapist. The occupational therapist is equally involved, being concerned with activities of daily living other than ambulation. Imagine such ordinary things as dressing, bathing, visiting the toilet, and many other activities all carried out by a normal individual without any thought. Consider the advanced age of many primary amputees and finally try bathing yourself or dressing yourself with only one leg supporting your weight. It may be humorous to the normal person, but certainly not so to the amputee. All of these matters are part of positive amputee rehabilitation and since they first become apparent in hospital, it is frequently the responsibility of the occupational therapist or nursing staff to recognise the need for advice and offer it when the occasion demands. This is all part of *total* patient care, an aspect of treatment which is tending to be lost in the present day plethora of super-specialisation.

Dressing can be eased in many ways. The prosthetic foot, being relatively rigid, may cause difficulty with trouser legs—for this reason most men remove limb and trousers at the same time. The PTB wearer, particularly in these days of changing fashion, is penalised if wearing 'drain pipe' fashions—then he must use a zip fastening stitched into the inner seam of the trouser leg. This eases application of the limb in the morning or changing of stump socks during the day, especially in warm weather.

Simple things like rising from a chair can be performed easily by the amputee if the correct technique is used. Various bathing aids may be necessary, certainly in the case of the bilateral lower limb amputee. He can be taught to transfer on his bottom from a wheelchair via a bath board and bath stool into the bath. Slippery bath surfaces are best dealt with by applying strips of Scotch Tread, an excellent and inexpensive way of ensuring greater safety. Patients can be assessed regarding the need for such things as grab rails in the bathroom, toilet, or house entrance. The possibilities are endless and staff frequently add suggestions which prove most useful, especially for the elderly. Assistance and advice must often be given to the patient who, following his discharge from the hospital, should continue to attend as an outpatient. It should be remembered that attendance must continue as long as the patient is ambulant, perhaps amounting to a lifetime. It may involve special interests normally associated with the different decades of life; the young child with rapidly changing interests and desires, the adolescent, and the various stages of adult life. All of these may require prosthetic adaptation to suit any particular activity of daily living. Thus the adolescent who seeks advice regarding sport, the father who may wish to go swimming with his young children, the older patient who may indulge in a great variety of activities, all need thoughtful consideration. One of the authors has knowledge of patients who have special skiing, swimming, and diving limbs. Even a 'dancing arm' has been supplied, the patient, a man in his forties being a keen amateur ballroom dancer requiring an artificial arm with the correct degree of forearm and wrist alignment and an acceptable cosmetic artificial hand. Another patient, who lost three limbs, works, drives a car, and swims as a hobby. Yet another, a young boy who lives on a farm, shoots and fishes despite the loss of an arm. The list could go on and so could the advice required in all of the many and varied pursuits.

The role of the occupational therapist normally continues in the patient's own home. The younger, active amputee will, of course, require no assistance of this type, but the elderly derive great benefit from adequate home assessment and adaptation. This, ideally, should be carried out prior to the patient's discharge from hospital and should involve an occupational therapist from the hospital service or one from the staff of the local Social Work Department. Each area has its own method of working but generally the end result is beneficial, making it possible for elderly patients to return to their own domestic surroundings. It is essential that the community occupational therapist is aware of the patient's ability and the degree to which rehabilitation has progressed. She is then in a position to give both practical help and encouragement in the new situation which must be faced.

The importance of a close link-up between the hospital and community services cannot be overestimated.

The Health Visitor should be notified long before the patient is ready for discharge home and should meet the patient and, if possible, the family. The case history should be known and future problems highlighted.

If the services of the community nurse are required a detailed transfer letter should be forwarded and arrangements can be made for the loan of equipment such as a bed cradle or commode.

Requests for a Home Help and for Meals on Wheels can be made to the Social Work Department. The provision of aids or services such as these may make all the difference to the elderly, allowing continued independence in the family home. Many of these aspects of total care are within the province of the occupational therapist—in a sense they are providing practical social welfare but more importantly they are promoting better communication, an essential aspect of this type of work. This interest extends into the home, rehousing at ground level perhaps being necessary for the double amputee. The provision of a wheelchair may be necessary and the door width measurements will be needed so that the correct size of wheelchair can be issued. For safety it should be a chair with an extended wheel base as the centre of gravity of the body moves back in a double amputee when seated and there is a danger of backward tipping of the chair.

The Disablement Resettlement Officer may be asked to interview an amputee regarding future employment and there can be the question of whether or not assessment at a government Skillcentre could prove useful. Assessment may indicate the need for retraining since there may be a complete incompatibility between the physical disability and normal employment. Employment may depend on the ability of the patient to use public transport but in double amputees mobility allowance may apply and in certain cases, e.g. War Pensioners, there may be eligibility for motorised transport.

The Technical Officer attached to Limb Fitting Centres is concerned with wheelchair provision and the provision of transport. He may also offer advice on adaptations necessary to normal controls of motorised vehicles.

It is true to say that what is observed may not always be understood. Hospital staff are trained observers and the importance of correct interpretation of what is seen cannot be overemphasised. Care of the amputee is an intensely human activity and staff involved in this work obtain a new perspective—perhaps this is because total care of the patient is their watchword. Independence is a human right. It is certainly the purpose of amputee rehabilitation and all treatment and management should be directed towards this end.

## Summary of occupational therapy

Categories of patients varying therapy:

1 single amputee,
2 double amputee,
3 high level single amputee,
4 amputee with concurrent disability.

Other factors causing variation:

1 age,
2 motivation,
3 mental status.

Basic areas of interest of therapist:

1 wheelchair training;
2 ADL
   (a) preprosthetic fitting,
   (b) postprosthetic fitting;

3 remedial activity
 (a) preprosthetic fitting,
 (b) postprosthetic fitting,
 (c) work assessment;

4 supportive treatment
 (a) social,
 (b) diversional.

**Wheelchair training—postoperative**

Offers immediate mobility
Offers remedial activity involving trunk and upper limbs
Accurate prescription necessary even for temporary use, e.g. wheelchair size, provision of stump rests, extended wheel base
Instruction in use of wheelchair-transfers:
 pivot with good leg
 sideways
 backwards/forwards
Instruction in use of wheelchair:
 push ups to ease seating pressure
 manoeuvring and general chair use
 ADL:
  dressing
  toileting
Permanent issue if
(a) prosthetic fitting impossible,
(b) double amputee.

If so check compatibility: wheelchair/patient/environment. May require further change in wheelchair prescription

**ADL (a) Preprosthetic fitting (single amputee)**

Transfers: wheelchair/bed/toilet/bath;
Rising:
 bed/walking aid
 chair/walking aid
 toilet/walking aid, and reverse
Self-care:
 dressing in bed;
 use of clothing adaptations, e.g. zips and velcro;
 use overhead grab rail;
 aid offered by rigid bedside cabinet for hand support;
 toileting, use of support hand rails and toilet raisers;
 washing,
 at basin in wheelchair;

bath transfers;
non-slip strips;
bathboard and/or stool;
'domestic' duties, washing small items of clothing, helping to set lunch tables, etc.

**ADL (b) Postprosthetic fitting**

More intensive
Domestic activities of primary importance
Educational activities of secondary importance
Work activities of secondary importance
Recreational activities of secondary importance
Home visit allows assessment
Identification hazards:
- rugs
- doorsills
- Suitability of seating
- Suitability of bed height
- Suitability of bed firmness
- Accessibility of kitchen equipment

Hand rails:
- steps
- stairs

Aid requirements
Contact with Community OT

**ADL (c) Preprosthetic fitting (double amputee)**

Sitting balance
Use of rope ladder attached to foot of bed
'Bottom' walking on firm bed
Transfers: usually forward/backward
Self-care: trousers and shirts applied on bed, side to side rocking allowing application of garment
Toilet:
- height to match wheelchair seating
- forward transfer with back to front toilet position
- toilet frame bolted to floor for hand support

Bathing: side transfers from wheelchair to bathboard and into bath via bath stool. Necessity for grab rails

**ADL (d) Postprosthetic fitting (double amputee)**

Independence determined by balance, standing tolerance, and reaching ability
Varying prosthetic/wheelchair use
Possible need for ramps
Possible need for adjustment kitchen
Work surfaces
Review of wheelchair prescription

**ADL (e) Special considerations for associated disability**

Diabetes:
- complication of reduced vision
- complication of peripheral neuropathy and alteration of sensation

Hemiplegia:
- special wheelchair propulsion
- hand/foot propulsion
- one handed training

Parkinsonism:
- effect on standing balance
- benefit of aids

Osteoarthritis:
- problem mainly one of standing up and sitting down
- chair height and design

Rheumatoid arthritis:
- aid dependent
- special problems with hand grip

Cardiorespiratory disability:
- well graded remedial activities in keeping with clinical presentation

**Remedial activity**

Upper limb strength:
- floor games
- wood work
- printing
- weaving

Sitting balance (double):
- floor games
- snooker
- therapeutic garden, etc.

Work assessment:
- use of remedial activities in making assessment
- contact with DRO

**Supportive treatment**

Recreation: very varied
Social activity: very varied
Diversional: very varied

**Home environment check list**

1 Doorway widths (particularly bathroom which is usually the narrowest)
2 Door opening—direction
3 Corridor widths and general lay out including corners
4 Steps/stairs—number and depth
5 Bed—height and firmness
6 Toilet—height and positioning
7 Bath—general dimensions
8 Chair—height seating and armrests
9 Kitchen—height units, working surfaces, cupboards; knee room for accessibility
10 General—height and position of switches, sockets, door handles, window catches; type of floor covering

# 16 Feelings, Failings, and Frustrations

The very young child who has undergone amputation for limb deformity or trauma will not be concerned about being different from other children as long as he is able to move around fairly quickly and play with his friends. His young playmates will tend to accept him as long as he can keep pace with them.

It is important, however, that the parents accept the child's disability, for occasions may arise when the child overhears some unwise remark or suffers teasing by other children. It is then that the child will need support and understanding and an explanation of why amputation was necessary.

When there is no urgency for amputation, e.g. in cases of limb discrepancy, it is essential to delay surgery until the youngster is old enough to take part in the discussions and make a decision. It is helpful if he can talk with a well established amputee so that the advantages and disadvantages of amputation can be better understood.

No teenager wishes to be singled out as different. If amputation has been done to remove a noticeably deformed leg the prosthesis will be accepted with relief and there will be an eagerness to be accepted as an equal among friends. The teenager wishes to be admired by the opposite sex; therefore it is of the utmost importance that prostheses have a good cosmetic appearance and allow a normal gait. Patients have been heard to remark: 'How nice to have a pair of feet that match'; the quality of life for these amputees becomes greatly improved since they no longer feel different. Psychologically they become well adjusted, accepting life as amputees far more readily than they accepted their early teenage years.

The young person who has had an amputation suddenly thrust on him (as a result of trauma) may abhor the mutilation his body has suffered and resent the change in visual appearance. There may be bitterness that this disaster has happened. There may be fear that the whole way of life will be altered and there may be anxiety regarding the future. This anxiety will be worse if there are family responsibilities. In the case of a man: will he be able to continue in his present job? Will his workmates consider he is now less capable than them? How will his family, especially his wife, react to his changed appearance? Will his children look upon him as different from other fathers? If the amputee is a woman, she will experience similar feelings and doubts. Perhaps cosmesis will colour these views.

The patient's sexuality need not change although one might reasonably presume that this is likely. The age groups involved are the young and middle aged and generally amputation is due to trauma, pre-existing deformity, or discrepancy. Any change is clearly allied to the patient's personality and any degree of extroversion either caused or exaggerated by the amputation is likely to increase the sexual activity. There is some evidence that this happens. The effect of amputation on the introverted individual is difficult to judge. Perhaps this aspect of total care is best defined by saying that it is extremely rare for a patient to seek advice and direct questioning infrequently reveals any problem. It may be that advice is sought from a general practitioner or other counsellor. The patient will wish to be treated by family and friends as before amputation. Excessive sympathy and emotion may cause embarrassment and there may be a dislike of being dependent on others. Early delivery of the prosthesis is essential not only in order to regain independence but also to restore body image.

On delivery of the prosthesis the patient will be eager to start walking again. This eagerness can be excessive and the patient may wish to attempt too high a level of activity too soon. It must be borne in mind that stump tissues are not physiologically suitable for weight bearing and too much early walking training may cause skin abrasions and a frustrating delay in progress.

By this time the patient should have begun to think positively about the future. Looking at the stump should no longer cause distress and washing and bandaging it should cause no problems. The stump should be recognised as the connecting link between the patient and the prosthesis.

No two people have the same emotional outlook. One with a well adapted personality will strive towards complete independence, will have self-confidence and will do well. Another may use the disability to avoid responsibilities and to gain sympathy. This type of patient will have many complaints and the prosthesis will never give satisfaction. There will be no hurry to return to work and the amputee will never be a successful prosthetic user. Fortunately this type of patient is in the minority.

The elderly amputee generally comes to amputation as a result of vascular disease, therefore there has been considerable pain during the preceding months, perhaps claudicating at first and rest pain later. The greatest desire is to be free from pain and the loss of a leg is accepted to obtain relief. There is usually worry about the ability to cope with the normal activities of everyday life afterwards. Since the spouse and friends are also elderly there may not be a great deal of help available.

Reassurance, encouragement, and an outline of the help available should be given. The patient's ability to comprehend and retain information is often limited and explanations regarding help need to be repeated more than once and should be made to the relatives as well. The rehabilitation programme should also be explained.

The elderly patient's postoperative feeling is one of relief that the matter has finally been decided and the change in visible appearance is not unduly worrying. However, a phantom limb, painless or otherwise, is very strange and may be difficult to accept.

Mental outlook depends to a great extent on home circumstances. If a welcome home is assured regardless of the functional ability, the patient will be content to take each day as it comes, gradually learning to become more mobile and more independent. If, on the other hand, the patient fears the possibility of being a burden to relatives there may be a feeling that life is really not worth living and the effort to achieve independence may not seem worthwhile.

Often the elderly amputee who lives alone is aware of the difficulty experienced moving about the home before operation and may wonder whether it will be feasible to live alone again following surgery. In all likelihood the patient will be quite satisfied to move quietly about his own home knowing a relative, neighbour, or home help can come in daily and that members of the Community Services can be contacted should more specialised assistance be needed.

Throughout, the amputee must have caring team support. The team must be professional in their approach—interdisciplinary consultation must take place at all times to achieve total care. The care must be positive—consultation is not merely a professional activity—it must include the patient who values communication, explanation, and the opportunity to raise any matter requiring further clarification.

# Glossary of Terms

**Abduction** Movement of a limb or stump outwards

**Abduction deformity** A stump positioned in abduction

**Ablation** Removal

**Above-knee amputation** An amputation between the hip and the knee

**Adduction** Movement of a limb or stump inwards

**Adduction deformity** A stump positioned in adduction

**Adductor roll** A roll of flesh not contained within the socket on the adductor or inner side of the socket brim

**Alignment jig** A device which allows variation in the alignment of a limb

**Anteroposterior** From front to back

**Below-knee amputation** An amputation between the knee and the ankle

**Bioengineering** The application of biomechanics

**Biomechanics** Concerns the application of mechanics to the human body

**Carbon fibre** A reinforcing material used in laminating sockets

**Claudication** Limp, usually referring to pain on walking

**Closed suction drainage** Drainage of a wound directly into a vacuumised container

**Concurrent disability** A disability existing at the same time

**Contralateral hand** The hand on the opposite side

**Cosmesis** Appearance of normality or that degree of normality achieved

**Definitive limb** One for permanent use fabricated according to a prescription designed around the patient's needs

**Distal** At the outer, further end, e.g. of a stump

**Dorsal** Pertaining to the back

**End bearing pad** A pad incorporated into a socket to accept the loading of an end bearing stump, e.g. a Syme's

**Epiphysis** The 'growing end' of a long bone

**Equinus** Forefoot, or stump in partial foot amputation, pointing down

**Eversion** Turning outwards, e.g. of the foot

**External rotation** Turning outwards, e.g. of the hip

**Feedback** Sensory appreciation of distal touch or pressure

**Female cast** A plaster cast of a stump which, when filled with liquid plaster, produces a male or positive model
**Filler** A material, often wood, simply to occupy space or create a shape
**Flexion deformity** A stump position in flexion
**Foot slap** Excessively heavy and rapid heel strike to foot flat action
**Functional splint** A splint which actively assists function
**Gait cycle** The sequence of events in taking a step
**Glass wool** Fibre glass wool used in limb fabrication
**Gritti–Stokes amputation** An amputation through the femoral condyles
**Hemiplegia** Paralysis, complete or partial, of one side of the body
**High loading** Excessive localised pressure
**Hindquarter amputation** An amputation at the hip and including the hemipelvis
**Hip disarticulation** An amputation through the hip joint
**Interface** The areas of direct surface contact, e.g. between the stump and the socket
**Inversion** Turning inwards, e.g. of the foot
**IPOF** Immediate postoperative fitting, e.g. of a plaster allowing early mobilisation
**Knee control** A mechanical device in a prosthesis to control the action of the knee joint
**Laminate** Materials bonded together
**Lateral** The outer aspect
**Low bed** A bed adjusted with the mattress at the same level as the wheelchair seating to assist in transfer
**Male model** A plaster replica produced from a plaster cast of a stump
**Moment** The tendency of a force to produce rotation
**Neuroma** The anatomical change in a nerve when cut
**Osteomyoplasty** A plastic operation involving muscle and bone, designed to reconstruct and restore function, e.g. in a stump
**Osteosarcoma** A malignant tumour of bone
**Patellar-tendon-bearing** A type of below-knee prosthesis
**Peg** A simple pylon support
**Pelvic band** A reinforced belt fastening around the pelvic brim aiding suspension and positioning of an above-knee prosthesis
**Physiological splint** A splint which positions a joint or joints to obtain maximum function
**Pistoning** An in and out movement of the stump in the socket
**Polyurethane end pad** A shaped pad produced in expanded polyurethane for the end of the stump
**Primary amputation** Amputation for the first time
**Prosthesis** A replacement part; in this context an artificial limb
**Prosthetist** A ‘limb fitter’ highly skilled in the fabrication, fitting, and alignment of artificial limbs
**Proximal** Nearer the trunk; as opposed to distal

**Push off** Forward propulsion when walking afforded by the toe just before it leaves the ground to enter the swing phase

**Rem–Daw sheath** A nylon under sock

**Rocker end** A rocker shaped 'foot' commonly used with a pylon limb

**Sach foot** Solid ankle cushion heel

**Sarcoma** A malignant tumour

**Side steels** A means of connecting one prosthetic component to another, e.g. a thigh to a shin

**Socket** The part of the prosthesis in contact with the stump

**Socket brim** The top brim of the socket

**Stance** The period of the gait cycle when the foot is in contact with the ground

**Suction socket** One in which suspension is achieved by creating an air seal at the socket and thus a negative pressure within, reducing the tendency of the stump to withdraw

**Suspension cuff** A leather cuff used to suspend the limb on the stump

**Swing** The period of the gait cycle when the foot is off the ground

**Syme's amputation** An amputation just above the ankle

**Thenar eminence** The base of the thumb

**Thigh corset** Produced in blocked leather, enclosing the thigh and incorporating side steels attached through a knee joint to the shin of the prosthesis

**Through-knee amputation** An amputation through the knee joint

**Vaulting** Excessive elevation of the pelvis on the support side during mid stance

# Bibliography

The 'Denny' Report *The Future of the Artifical Limb Service in Scotland.* (Report of a Working Party set up by the Secretary of State for Scotland) 1970

Friedmann, L W (1978) *The Psychological Rehabilitation of the Amputee.* Springfield, Illinois, Charles C. Thomas

Humm, W (1977) *Rehabilitation of the Lower Limb Amputee* (Third Edition). London, Baillière Tindall

Little, J M (1975) *Major Amputations for Vascular Disease.* Edinburgh, London, and New York, Churchill Livingstone

McKibbin, B (ed) (1975) *Recent Advances in Orthopaedics* (Number 2). Edinburgh, London, and New York, Churchill Livingstone

Murdoch, G (ed) (1970) *Prosthetic and Orthotic Practice*; based on a Conference held in Dundee, June 1969. London, Arnold

Vitali, M, Robinson, K P, Andrews, B G and Harris, E E (1978) *Amputations and Prostheses.* London, Baillière Tindall

# Index


Alignment, 80, 100
  jig, 81
Amputation
  above-knee, 34, 49, 62
  below-knee, 38, 50, 63
  Chopart, 51
  Gritti–Stokes, 37
  hindquarter, 34, 48, 62
  hip disarticulation, 34, 48
  indications for, 24
  levels of, 34–39
  limiting factors in, 34–39
  Lisfranc, 51
  partial foot, 39–51
  surgery, 47–51
  Syme's, 39, 50, 65
  through-knee, 37, 49, 63
  toes, 51
  transmetatarsal, 51
Amputee
  double, 55, 58, 92, 112, 120
  elderly, 126
  teenager, 125
  young, 125
Antibiotics, 43, 44
Aortography, 43
Arteriography, 43
Artificial Limb Service, 4
Atheroma, 24, 25
Atherosclerosis—see Vascular disease

Bandages, crêpe, 61
Bandaging, 58, 61, 71–75
Bathing aids, 54–56, 118
Bioengineer, 17, 52
Bone, medulla of, 49

Callosities, 78
Chair
  rising from, 111
  sitting down on, 109
Chondrosarcoma, 48
Complications, postoperative, 58–60
Confusional state, 58
Controlled environment treatment, 68–70
Cosmesis, 28, 38, 39
Counselling, 40

Denny Report, 4
Dermatitis, contact, 78
Diabetes mellitus, 24, 25, 40, 42, 50, 57
Diet, 42, 57
Disablement Resettlement Officer, 120
Doppler methods, 44

Embolic impaction, 24
Embolism, pulmonary, 58
Energy, 17, 18
Epidermoid cysts, 78
Exercises
  bed, 104
  resisted, 104

Fairing, 87
Flexion deformity, 34, 36, 38, 46, 100, 104
Floor, rising from, 111
Foot, contralateral, care of, 42, 57
Force, 17, 18

Gait
  abnormalities of, 99–103
  normal, 6, 17–23
Gait training, 116
Gravity, 17, 18
  centre of, 18, 22

Haematoma, 58, 78
Health Visitor, 119
Heel strike, 21
Heparin, mini, 44, 58
Home assessment, 119

Immediate postoperative fitting (IPOF), 65–67
Infection, 2
  chest, 58

chronic, 24, 47
control of, 43
Insulin, 42, 57
International Society for Prosthetics and Orthotics, 5
Intertrigo, 78
Isotope clearance, 44

Joints,
ankle, 12
forefoot, 14
hip, 6
knee, 8

Knee, retention of, 38, 47

Limb
Anglesey, 2
deficiency classification, 31–32
deficiency, congenital, 24, 30
deformity, 24, 28, 47, 50
discrepancy, 24, 28, 47, 50
phantom, 57, 79
preparation for surgery, 44

Medical procedures, 43
Medical Social Worker, 40, 46, 52
Mobility aid, pneumatic, postamputation (PPAM aid), 106
Modular assembly systems, 85, 87
Moment, 17
Muscles
ankle-joint, 13–15
forefoot, 14
groups of, 7, 40
hip, 7–10
knee-joint, 9–12

Nerve, division of, 49
Neuroma, 49, 78, 79, 100
Nurse, 40, 52
community, 119
Nursing area, 52

Occupational therapist, 40, 52
therapy, 46, 118–124
Oscillometry, 43
Osteoclastoma, 48
Osteomyelitis, 28
Osteosarcoma, 26, 34, 48

Pain
burning, 41
claudicating, 25
phantom, 79
relief of, 41, 56, 57
stump, 77, 78
throbbing, 41
Paralysis, 28
Periosteal tube, 50
Physiotherapist, 40, 52
Physiotherapy, 46, 104–117
Plethysmography, 43
Poliomyelitis, 28
Postoperative care, 52–58
Povidone–iodine, 44
Preoperative care, 40–46
Prosthesis
above-knee, 83, 90
below-knee, 84, 94–96
care of, 98
Fajal, 94
Fillauer, 94
partial-foot, 85
patellar-tendon-bearing, 94
Syme's, 84, 96–97
temporary, 90, 115
through-hip, 82, 90
through-knee, 83, 93
Prosthetic replacement, 80–89
Prosthetist, 4, 40, 52, 81

Rehabilitation, 118–124
Rehabilitation specialist, 52
Rem–Daw sheath, 60
Rocker pylons, 112
application of, 92

Scar, adherent, 60
Sequestrum formation, 60
Skin flaps, 49, 50
Social Work Department, 119
Stairs
ascending, 111
descending, 112
Stance phase, 20
Steinmann's pins, 51
Stump
care of, 76
function of, 76
healed, the, 70
tremor, 57
socks, 90
Stump dressings
soft, 61, 62
elasticated adhesive, 61
rigid, 51, 61–68
Sutures, removal of, 62
Swing phase, 21

Team approach, 4, 40, 52, 127

Technical Officer, 120
Thermography, 44
Thrombosis, deep venous, 104
Thrombus formation, 24
Trauma, 27, 50, 125
Tumour, 26, 48

Vascular disease, 3, 24, 40, 42, 46, 47, 50
  pathology of, 24

Walking frame, 108
  rails, 104, 107
  sticks, 107
  sticks, Fischer, 108
Wheelchair, 55, 120
Wound
  breakdown, 60
  drainage, 77
  infection, 59